A Smart Woman's Guide
to Heart Health
...And the Hearts of the Men They Love

A Smart Woman's Guide to Heart Health

...And the Hearts of the Men They Love

Lorna Vanderhaeghe, M.S.
with Michelle Hancock, M.J.
Fitness by Byron Collyer, BSc. HKIN

Fitzhenry & Whiteside

Fitzhenry and Whiteside Limited
195 Allstate Parkway
Markham, Ontario L3R 4T8

In the United States:
311 Washington Street,
Brighton, Massachusetts 02135

www.fitzhenry.ca   godwit@fitzhenry.ca

Fitzhenry & Whiteside acknowledges with thanks the Canada Council for the Arts,
and the Ontario Arts Council for their support of our publishing program.
We acknowledge the financial support of the Government of Canada through
the Book Publishing Industry Development Program (BPIDP) for our publishing activities.

**Canada Council
for the Arts**

**Conseil des Arts
du Canada**

ONTARIO ARTS COUNCIL
CONSEIL DES ARTS DE L'ONTARIO

Library and Archives Canada Cataloguing in Publication
Vanderhaeghe, Lorna R.
A smart woman's guide to heart health : and the hearts of the men they love /
Lorna Vanderhaeghe, Michelle Hancock.
"Heart fitness by Byron Collyer."
Includes bibliographical references and index.
ISBN 978-1-55455-157-6
1. Heart diseases in women—Prevention—Popular works.
2. Heart diseases in women—Popular works. I. Hancock, Michelle,
1974- II. Title.
RC672.V36 2010   616.1'205082   C2010-900589-9

United States Cataloguing-in-Publication Data
Vanderhaeghe, Lorna.
A smart woman's guide to heart health : and the hearts of the men they love
Lorna Vanderhaeghe ; Michelle Hancock.
[304] p. : cm.
Summary: A safe and effective program for heart disease prevention and treatment.
ISBN: 978-1-55455-157-6 (pbk.)
1. Heart diseases in women — Popular works. 2. Women's health — Popular works.
I. Hancock, Michelle. II. Title.
616.1/20082 dc22   RC682.V363 2010

Note: If you are taking prescription medications, consult your physician before applying the recommendations
in the book. If you are taking Coumadin or Warfarin, you should not change your diet, add any new drugs either
over-the-counter or prescription, or add any new supplements without consulting your physician.

Disclaimer: This publication contains the opinions and ideas of its authors and is designed to provide useful
advice in regard to the subject matter covered. The authors and publisher are not engaged in rendering medical,
therapeutic, or other professional services in this publication. This publication is not intended to provide a
basis for action in particular circumstances without consideration by a competent professional. The authors
and publisher expressly disclaim any responsibility for any liability, loss, or risk, personal or otherwise, which is
incurred as a consequence, directly or indirectly, of the use and application of any of the contents of this book.

BMI Chart on page 36 reprinted from *The Body Sense Natural Diet: Six Weeks to a Slimmer, Healthier You* by Lorna
Vanderhaeghe courtesy of John Wiley & Sons Canada, Ltd.

Printed in Canada

We dedicate this book to the women and men
who have bravely faced cardiovascular disease;

To the researchers and health-care providers
who are changing the way we treat heart disease;

And, most importantly, to prevention
of the number one killer of North Americans.

Thank you to all of the men and women who have shared their health challenges and are seeking vibrant health. Your stories are the basis for each of my books. Most of all, to my family — Crystal, Kevin, Kyle, Caitlyn, Max, Finn, Connor and my five grandchildren — you are the reason I work tirelessly for better health care for all. To my lover and best friend Trevor — your love gives me the strength to pursue my dreams.

To Michelle Hancock — you are an amazing person. To Byron Collyer, who not only wrote the fitness section but has also whipped my body into shape — thank you for your contribution. To Allison Ross, who is so incredibly fit — thank you for allowing us to photograph you for the fitness section. My longtime friends John Morgenthaler, Ronald Reichert and Anthony Almada — your research expertise and friendship are invaluable. To Karlene Karst and Sherry Torkos — thank you for your steadfast support and loyalty when I needed it the most. To Dean Mosca, my caring friend and colleague — without you, this book would not have been born.

Contents

INTRODUCTION 1

1. ALL ABOUT THE HEART 5
   Heart and Arteries: Friends for Life 6
   One Powerful Pump 7
   Our Artery Helpers 8
   Clogged Pipes 9
   The Role of Cholesterol 9
   Free Radicals and Antioxidants. 12
   When Plaque Ruptures 13
   Other Heart Conditions 14
        Arrhythmias 14
        Valve Disorders 15
        Heart Failure. 16

2. HEART DISEASE RISKS 19
   Age 19
   Gender 20
   Low Thyroid and Hormones 20
   The Truth about HRT and Heart Disease 21
   Estrogen Does Not Predict Heart Disease Risk. 22
        The Coronary Drug Project 23
        The HERS Trial 24
        The PHASE Study. 25
        The WHI Study. 26
        The PEPI Trial and Bioidentical Progesterone 27
   What Is a Woman to Do?. 27
   HRT — Calcium and Magnesium 29
   Family History 32
   Smoking 33
   Obesity 34
   Inactivity 37

3. THE LOWDOWN ON CHOLESTEROL AND HIGH BLOOD PRESSURE..39
    Good Cholesterol 41
    Triglycerides. 42
    Lipoprotein(a) and Apolipoprotein B 43
    Homocysteine: Too Much of a Good Thing 44
    High Iron: Dangerous. 45
    Fibrinogen: Blood Clot Indicator 45
    C-reactive Protein: Inflammation Agent. 47
    High Blood Pressure (Hypertension) .50
        Systolic vs. Diastolic 50

4. DIABETES AND DEPRESSION: DOUBLE TROUBLE 53
    Steady Sugar Destruction 53
    Not Sweet for the Heart 54
    Sugar Speeds Aging 55
    Lifestyle Is the Best Drug. 56
    Diabetes Prevention 56
    The Adrenal Connection 57
    Heart Disease Linked to Depression .60
    Women More At Risk 61
    Achy, Breaky Heart 61
    Formulate Your Heart Health Plan. .62
    Lifesaving Support 62
    Anger Hurts the Heart 63
    Anxiety – The False Heart Attack 65

5. HEART-SMARTEN UP ON CARBS AND FATS. 67
    What Is a Carbohydrate? 67
        Food Glycemic Index 70
        The Low-Glycemic Solution. 71
    Hearts Love Fiber. 72
    Fat Phobia 73
    Saturated Fats. 74
    The Coconut Truth 75
    The Deadliest Fats. 77
    Unsaturated Fats: Not Just Good but Fabulous. 78
    Why We Need Essential Fats. 78

Omega-3 Superstars.................................79
Mercury Hinders the Heart 81
Echium: A Premium Heart Oil.........................82
Echium Fights Inflammation..........................84

6. EAT THE HEART-HEALTHY WAY............................87
Protein Provides Power 87
The Protein Difference..............................89
The Soy Story......................................91
Calcium Can Clog Arteries...........................92
Eat Like a Mediterranean............................93
Preserve Heart Longevity............................94
Powerful Pomegranate...............................95
Dangerously Sugary Drinks...........................97
Caffeine in a Cup 97
The Sodium-Potassium Connection....................99
Pumping Up Potassium 100
Mighty Magnesium 101
Multipurpose Heart Mineral 102

7. HEART HEALTH PERSONAL ASSESSMENT....................105
How Did You Score? 108

8. HEART-HEALTHY RECIPES...............................109
Getting Started 109
No Fake Sweeteners 111
More Heart Health Cooking Tips 112
        Breakfast..................................119
        Appetizers, Dips, and Snacks...............123
        Dressings 129
        Salads 131
        Soupy Stuff 137
        Vegetables.................................145
        Main Dishes 150
        Condiments 155
        Desserts and Baked Stuff...................158
        Spreads & Egg Replacement 163

9. HEART-HEALTHY NUTRIENTS 165
    Sytrinol Lowers Cholesterol and Triglycerides in 30 Days . .166
        Sytrinol Keeps Arteries Clear. 166
        Sytrinol Is a Powerful Antioxidant 167
        Sytrinol Improves Your LDL:HDL Ratio 167
        Sytrinol's Five Actions Maintain a Healthy Heart 169
    Pycnogenol Protects the Heart. 172
        Pycnogenol Lowers High Blood Pressure 173
        Pycnogenol – Blood Clot Preventer. 174
        Pycnogenol Repairs Capillaries. 174
        Pycnogenol Prevents Fat Deposition in Artery Walls . .174
    Coenzyme Q10 – The Heart Superstar 175
        Statin Drugs Deplete Q10 175
        Statins Increase Breast Cancer Risk. 176
        CoQ10 Lowers Blood Pressure. 177
        Cardiovascular Benefits of CoQ10 177
    Marvelous Magnesium. 179
        Potassium and Sodium Need Magnesium 179
        Magnesium Protects Against Stroke 179
        Magnesium Lowers Bad Cholesterol
            While Increasing Good. 180
        Magnesium Regulates Blood Pressure 181
    Multivitamins and Minerals to the Rescue. 181
    Niacin – Proven Cholesterol-busting Vitamin. 183
        Non-flushing Niacin for Intermittent Claudication. . . .184
        Non-flushing Niacin Lowers Fibrinogen 184
    Heart Health Nutrient Program 185

10. HEART HEALTH FITNESS TRAINING 187
    Weights: Invaluable for Heart Health 187
    Equipment 190
    Core Training Tips for Your Program 191
    Program Outline 193
    Warm-up (every day) 194
    Conclusion 217

11. HOW TO TAME STRESS. 219
     Fight or Flight: Our Genetic Legacy. 220
     Why We Need to Relax 221
     Anti-stress Strategies. 224
         Deep Breathing 224
         Yoga: Ancient Practice Has Heart. 227
         Meditate Stress Away. 229
         Simple Meditation Exercise 230

12. THINK HAPPY, LIVE WITH HEART 233
     Healing Heart Visualization. 235
     Do You Live with Heart? 236
     Have a Positive Outlook. 237
     Laughter: The Best Medicine?. 239
     Self-honesty: Emotions and Expression 241
     Final Cardio Sense. 244
     A Heart Health Conclusion 246

REFERENCES AND RESOURCES 249

INDEX 263

A Smart Woman's Guide
to Heart Health

Introduction

*"Educating the mind without educating
the heart is no education at all."*
— Aristotle

Nobody suspected Grandma Ruby had heart problems until she collapsed on Christmas Day while preparing dinner. To her family and friends, she'd always seemed invincible. A tireless housekeeper never without a dishcloth in her hands or a leaf blower hoisted on her back. A seasoned cook who spoiled guests with enough food to feed half the neighborhood. Even Ruby might not have suspected she had heart disease, a condition that affects millions and millions of North Americans. With her hardworking, old-school mentality, Ruby probably would have treated symptoms like breathlessness and tightness in the chest as an annoyance, a burden to bear, something not even worth a trip to the doctor. Tragically, had she sought help earlier and taken more proactive measures, Ruby probably would have lived past her mid-seventies.

There is a Grandma Ruby in everybody's life — a best friend, a co-worker, a partner, a cousin, or a sibling who has heart disease. In fact, heart disease afflicts one in three Americans. A heart attack or stroke kills someone every seven minutes in Canada.

Incredibly, the bulk of these deaths are women. And did you know our chance of being struck down by heart disease increases as we age? Today, women are more likely to die of a heart attack than of breast cancer — a surprising fact to many.

Cardiovascular disease (CVD) is an umbrella term for diseases and injuries of the heart (including valve and rhythm issues), heart failure, diseases of the blood vessels, and stroke. And for decades, the mental image of a red-faced man clutching his chest has dominated the media. However, we are now realizing — and publicizing — that due to a variety of factors, women are just as vulnerable as men to diseases of the cardiovascular system.

Startling Statistics

- Every 37 seconds, an American dies of cardiovascular disease (CVD)
- About 80,000,000 American adults (one in three) have one or more types of CVD
- Every 7 minutes, someone in Canada dies from heart disease or stroke
- Cardiovascular disease accounts for one-third of Canadian deaths
- About 70,000 heart attacks occur each year in Canada, resulting in 19,000 deaths

Over the past decade, the number of heart attack-related hospitalizations has risen steadily. And the personal costs are tremendous. For those who survive, heart disease can be a debilitating condition, affecting relationships and quality of life to deep degrees.

Although heart disease is a leading killer, there is an upside: it is preventable — and reversible. Like other progressive diseases such as diabetes and cancer, heart disease doesn't have to result in millions of patients who clutter hospitals, fill drug prescriptions, and require expensive operations. No matter what our age, regardless of whether we are 19 or 90, we can strengthen our hearts. We have the power within ourselves to make educated choices about diet, lifestyle, exercise, and supplements, and our bodies will reward us with disease-free vitality.

Diet is the first pillar of heart health. Well, maybe "diet" is the wrong word. Diet implies changing our eating habits for a designated period of time. Eating for our heart means making long-term changes to what's on our plate and in our glass. You do not want to be like most people who change their diet only upon diagnosis of a disease. Be proactive. By eating the Heart-Healthy way, you will not only help your heart, you will also provide your body with the nutrients and protective elements it needs to prevent and alleviate other degenerative ailments.

Related to diet is nutritional supplementation. Is supplementing really necessary, you might ask, if you are already doing everything else? The answer is a resounding "yes." Specific nutrients have been shown to have a markedly beneficial effect on ailing hearts, high cholesterol, and blood pressure. Even late-stage heart disease and post-surgery conditions can benefit from vitamins, minerals, and nutrients such as magnesium, coenzyme Q10, sytrinol, pycnogenol, and essential fatty acids.

Physical activity is another big component of any heart health program. A sedentary lifestyle weakens the heart and disrupts blood sugar levels, immunity, mental health and hormones. Conversely, getting fit is the cheapest and most effective therapy for overall health improvement. We will cover all this in Chapters 9 and 10.

No heart book is complete without discussion of stress reduction and management. Many risk factors for heart disease are exacerbated by stress. Stress itself is toxic for the heart. Related to stress is anxiety. Often panic attacks are mistaken for heart attacks, highlighting this very fundamental connection. There are various anti-stress and mental/emotional health strategies that play a valuable role in heart disease prevention and treatment.

Your heart will thank you for picking up this book because it means you want to make life changes. Maybe you have recently received a diagnosis you do not like. Maybe your cholesterol readings have been climbing for years but now they are dangerously high. Maybe you have a strong family history of heart disease that you want to avoid. It's never too early, or too late, to think about how to strengthen your hard-working heart. By combining a heart-healthy diet and key nutritional supplements with exercise and stress reduction strategies, you will quickly begin to strengthen and protect your heart.

1. All About the Heart

"The best and most beautiful things in this world cannot be seen or even heard, but must be felt with the heart."
— Helen Keller

If you turn on the TV, women in red dresses fill the screen. Some of them we recognize from magazines. Others are from our favorite sitcoms. Still others are the plain Janes who live next door and who could be any one of us. They are the new faces of heart disease. Not new in the sense that heart disease is new. It definitely is not. What is new about awareness campaigns like this one is the fact that they actually exist. Ten years ago, those red dresses were still hanging in the closet. But today, something has changed to bring heart disease to the forefront of public attention.

Women have lower rates of cardiovascular disease than men until age 40 (16 percent for men versus 8 percent for women). From ages 40 to 80, the rates for both sexes level off at roughly 73 percent. But by the time we reach 80, the cardiovascular disease rate for women surpasses that of men by 7 percent (86 and 79 percent, respectively). Much of this data comes from the well-known Framingham Heart Study by the National Heart, Blood and Lung Institute, which also indicated that the lifetime risk for cardiovascular disease is two in three for men, and more than one in two for women.

The mortality rate for heart disease, meanwhile, is just as staggering. Every year since 1900, except for 1918, cardiovascular disease has accounted for more deaths than any other single cause or group of causes of death in the U.S. In fact, cardiovascular disease claims the same number of lives every year as cancer, chronic lower respiratory diseases, accidents, and diabetes mellitus combined. In other words, it is the underlying cause (including congenital cardiovascular defects) for 35 percent of all deaths.

That is right. Every one in three deaths is contributable to a preventable condition that we can avoid by making heart-healthy choices.

We previously mentioned the Framingham Heart Study (FHS), which has been a huge source of information about disease incidence and heart disease risk factors. (It was, incidentally, one of the first heart studies to include women as well.) Prior to 1948, when the study began, doctors actually believed that blood pressure is supposed to rise as people age. Narrowing of the arteries (known as atherosclerosis and caused by the buildup of fatty tissue in artery walls) was thought to be inevitable. That view would change.

In Framingham, Massachusetts, more than 5,200 men and women between ages 30 and 62 enrolled in the study, underwent expansive tests, completed extensive medical questionnaires, and had their health re-tested over several two-year periods. There were later two subsequent studies including minorities and the children of the original participants. And in 2002, grandchildren of the original participants were enrolled to enter a new phase of this ongoing research project. What the researchers continue to uncover from the FHS and other large-scale investigations like it is a better biological understanding of how high cholesterol and high blood pressure, plus other factors — e.g., smoking, a sedentary lifestyle, and obesity — contribute to the development of heart disease. No doubt, 20 years from now we will look back and marvel again at how fast this knowledge has evolved. Still, one thing will not change: heart disease is a condition requiring a whole body and spirit approach to prevention and treatment.

Heart and Arteries: Friends for Life
The abundance of terms related to heart disease can get confusing. As we have mentioned, heart disease is not just one condition. Lots of cardiovascular problems affect not only the heart's ability to function well but also the blood vessels running throughout the body, which is why we often see cardiovascular issues in the brain, lungs, and lower

extremities, too. Cardiovascular disease is an umbrella term for heart disease (including valve and rhythm issues), heart failure, diseases of the blood vessels, and stroke. Coronary artery disease is by far the most common type of cardiovascular disease. Coronary artery disease is technically a disease of the arteries, the passageways that deliver — and restrict, if blocked — blood to the needy heart muscle. This disease often results in chest pain (angina) and heart attack. Another term you will often hear in this context is ischemic heart disease, which involves insufficient blood and oxygen flow to the body's tissues.

One Powerful Pump

Clench your fist and there you have the approximate shape and size of your heart muscle, nestled in behind your breastbone. The heart has four chambers — two upper (atria) and two lower (ventricles). Oxygen-depleted, bluish blood that has returned through the body collects in the right atrium, then flows down into the right ventricle. From there, it is pumped via the pulmonary artery to the lungs, where it picks up fresh oxygen. The now re-oxygenated, bright-red blood travels through the pulmonary veins back into the heart, but this time, it flows into the left atrium, and then down into the left ventricle. Finally, it leaves the heart through the aorta to begin its next cycle throughout the body.

What a process! The heart beats an average 100,000 times a day. Day in, day out, from birth to death (upward of 2.5 billion heartbeats), it delivers oxygen, nutrients, hormones, and other important constituents to every cell in our body. At the same time, the blood collects cellular junk — the unwanted waste of regular processes that occur inside cells. Think of this mighty heart muscle as the pump that keeps everything else running. Just like a mechanical pump needs fuel to keep working, the heart requires a steady supply of blood and oxygen to stay healthy. Problems arise when it does not get this fuel because somewhere in the system, a blockage has occurred.

Arteriosclerosis vs. Atherosclerosis

What is the difference between arteriosclerosis and atherosclerosis? They both relate to arteries, but arteriosclerosis is any process that causes damage and hardening/thickening of our major arteries. Atherosclerosis is the most common form of arteriosclerosis and specifically involves the buildup of artery-toughening plaque. When plaque buildup happens in the coronary arteries, we get heart disease. When it happens in other parts of the body, we get impaired circulation that can cause strokes, blood clots, and leg problems involving poor circulation, ulcers, poor wound healing, and gangrene.

Our Artery Helpers

The heart has two major arteries: the right coronary artery and the left main coronary artery. Each of these arteries stretches out into smaller and smaller arteries, delivering blood deeper into the heart muscle cells. If the blockage develops in one of these arteries, we call it atherosclerosis, from the Greek *athere*, meaning "porridge," and *sclerosis*, meaning "hardening" or "scarring." Over time, plaque builds on the arterial walls and causes them to stiffen. This accumulation narrows the arteries, and blood clots sometimes form on top of the plaque. The result is reduced blood flow through the heart. If blood flow stops completely, a heart attack (or myocardial infarction, meaning "death of heart tissue") occurs.

By far, the most common reason for reduced blood flow to the heart is atherosclerosis. However, there are other possible reasons for blocked arteries. Blood could be too thick, for instance. Ideally, blood is thin so it can pass unheeded through increasingly miniscule passageways on its way to and from cells. Sometimes, red blood cells have to bend and squeeze through single file because the arterial tunnel is so tiny! But when we, for example, eat too much fatty food, that fat ends up in the blood and clogs it up. Blood thickens and the cells also clump together if the body's clotting factors are affected. Our poor circulation then slows and the heart, meanwhile, is forced to work harder to counteract the effects of fatty blood.

Sometimes, the reason behind diminished blood flow lies with the heart muscle itself. Maybe it has been weakened or damaged from a previous heart attack. Or maybe the left ventricle, which pumps freshly oxygenated blood back into the body, has been damaged by high blood pressure. The left ventricle is particularly relevant to heart disease. Uncontrolled high blood pressure can cause poor left ventricle function and worsen heart disease.

Clogged Pipes

Far from being an inanimate pipe, our arteries are very much a player in this inner game of life. They, in fact, contract and expand in response to pressure.

Arteries have three layers, the outer, tougher adventitia; the middle smooth muscle media; and an inner layer (intima) that is lined with a single layer of specialized cells called the endothelium. This last ultra-thin barrier is a key component in the development of atherosclerosis.

Besides their ability to gauge blood pressure and flow, these multi-functioning endothelial cells interact with substances carried by blood, produce compounds that affect cell growth, and help govern muscle tone, thus allowing arteries to expand and contract. This expansion and contraction of arteries pushes blood along to where it is needed. Unfortunately, the endothelium layer frequently gets injured. The possible causes are many, including physical force and high blood pressure. Blood also carries toxins (environmental, dietary, metabolic), fatty proteins, excess blood sugar (glucose), infectious microbes, and unhealthy cholesterol. All of these can cause endothelial dysfunction and trigger the chain of events leading to atherosclerosis, high blood pressure, heart attack, stroke, and heart failure.

The Role of Cholesterol

Cholesterol has gotten a bad rap. Our bodies produce cholesterol — a waxy, fatty substance — which performs a number of important functions.

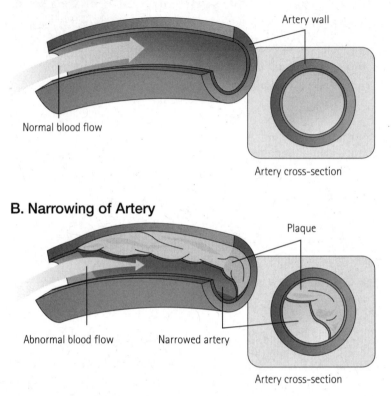

A. Normal Artery

Artery wall

Normal blood flow

Artery cross-section

B. Narrowing of Artery

Plaque

Abnormal blood flow   Narrowed artery

Artery cross-section

A. A NORMAL ARTERY   B. AN ARTERY CLOGGED WITH PLAQUE

Cholesterol is the building block of cellular membranes and is needed to make bile acids so we can digest and absorb our food. It is also needed to make vitamin D and hormones.

To move through the bloodstream, cholesterol puts on a protective coat of lipoprotein particles: low-density lipoprotein (LDL), the "bad" cholesterol, and high-density lipoprotein (HDL), the "good" cholesterol. Generally, we want to keep LDL cholesterol levels down to prevent it from lodging in arterial walls. Conversely, we want higher levels of HDL cholesterol, which protects the heart by sweeping LDL cholesterol through the arteries toward the liver. Here it is processed, then excreted from our system.

Dietary vs. Blood Cholesterol

Have you ever been told to avoid eggs because they are a "high cholesterol" food? This advice stems from a misunderstanding about the difference between dietary cholesterol and blood cholesterol. Dietary cholesterol is found in food, whereas blood cholesterol is made by the body and found in the bloodstream. Eating foods containing dietary cholesterol, however, will not necessarily put cholesterol into the bloodstream. Blood cholesterol is made in the liver from fats, sugars, and proteins, and the more processed foods and refined oils and sugars you consume, the more cholesterol is produced. Free-radical damage also causes the body to produce more cholesterol because cholesterol is used to repair damaged cells, tissues, and organs.

Studies show that eggs will not increase cholesterol levels but in fact may actually help lower them. Eggs contain lecithin, which emulsifies the cholesterol in them. Homogenized milk does more damage to arteries than eggs ever will because the fat globules in it have been mechanically altered to such a small state that they can be absorbed directly into the bloodstream.

A low-glycemic, unprocessed, healthy-fat diet is key to cholesterol reduction, and fiber is absolutely critical as it locks onto excess cholesterol and helps eliminate it. For diet recommendations, see Chapters 5 and 6.

When endothelial cells are damaged, they trigger an immune response. The body sends in a repair team to address the inflamed injury, but other scroungers also show up: blood fats and bad LDL cholesterol. Now, rather than help with repairs, immune cells begin an overzealous inflammatory process. As they migrate into the artery wall to help the injury, they ingest the LDL cholesterol and form bloated, fatty foam cells that end up forming atherosclerotic plaque. The damage is worse if the LDL cholesterol is oxidized, i.e., previously damaged by free radicals. Oxidized LDL cholesterol also damages neighboring cells at the injury site in a chain-reaction-type effect.

Free Radicals and Antioxidants

Think of rust for a minute. Slowly, various chemical reactions occur, resulting in an invasive corrosion that is the bane of every vehicle owner's existence! The damage created by free radicals in the body is like rust.

Free radicals are a natural byproduct of everyday reactions that produce energy for the body. Other major sources and generators include:

- Eating fried foods and heated oils
- Eating nitrates and nitrites in meats
- Toxic airborne chemicals
- Cigarette smoke, or smoke from forest fires
- Exposure to medical or electromagnetic radiation (i.e., computer terminals)
- Excessively strenuous exercise
- Drinking chlorinated water
- Eating a high-fat diet
- Prolonged physical and/or emotional stress

What these tiny molecules lack in size, they make up in destructive capacity. Many free radicals are highly toxic, mutagenic (cause cells to mutate), and carcinogenic (cause cancer). Stable molecules are held together by two electrons, but free radicals are missing one electron that they attempt to steal from neighboring molecules. Such molecular theft causes an undesirable ripple effect where other molecules in cells and cell membranes are damaged and more free radicals are formed. Eventually, if left unattended, what was once comparable to a spot of rust becomes a car riddled with unsightly holes.

The progression of free-radical damage can, fortunately, be kept in check with antioxidants from our food and nutritional supplements. Antioxidants are free-radical scavengers. They readily disable free radicals, preventing healthy body tissues from being damaged. When the body is deficient in antioxidants, our risk of disease increases and aging accelerates. By eating foods rich in antioxidants such as vitamins A, C, and E, selenium, and phytochemicals (the pigments that give plants their colors), we can keep our defenses against free radicals strong and stave off their heart-unfriendly effects. Supplemental pycnogenol, sytrinol, and coenzyme Q10 serve the same important function and further protect against heart disease via mechanisms that we will discuss later.

When Plaque Ruptures

As atherosclerosis progresses, arterial plaque grows and hardens as more cholesterol is absorbed into the artery wall along with other fats and inflammatory cells. A kind of cap forms over this. Some are big, some are small. Smaller plaques are more dangerous because they have a greater tendency to rupture in response to a variety of physical and emotional triggers. When this plaque ruptures, the immune system erroneously orders the production of factors that dissolve the plaque cap, causing its contents to spill back into the artery. Another immune response kicks in, attracting blood platelets. They clump together around the ruptured plaque and, along with red blood cells and other clotting factors, form a blood clot. If that blood clot fully blocks a coronary artery, a heart attack results.

How tragic that the first symptom of heart disease to be taken seriously is usually a heart attack and, sometimes, death!

The problem often lies in our general disconnect from our bodies. We are under such stressors in daily life that we miss or disregard many of the warning signs like chest pain, which occurs when coronary arteries narrow by about 50 percent. Medically termed angina (Latin for "squeezing of the chest") symptoms include:

- Pain radiating from the chest that spreads to your left arm, neck, back, throat, or jaw
- Tightness, pressure, squeezing, and/or aching in your chest or arm(s)
- Persistent sensation of moderate to severe indigestion

- Sharp, burning or cramping pain
- An ache starting in, or spreading to, your neck, jaw, throat, shoulder, back, or arm(s)
- Neck or upper back discomfort, particularly between the shoulder blades
- Numbness in your arms, shoulders, or wrists

Women with angina are more likely to notice abdomen, shoulder, and back discomfort than men. Likewise with actual heart attacks, symptoms vary between the sexes.

In the case of a heart attack or symptoms leading up to it, the quicker medical attention is sought, the greater the chances of avoiding heart damage. The longer blood supply is impeded or cut off, the more damage the heart potentially sustains. After 20 to 40 minutes, damage can be irreversible. Living tissue becomes scar tissue. Sadly, women are more likely to brush off bouts of warning signs, perhaps fearing embarrassment. When women do get a diagnosis and treatment, it usually occurs when they are older and heart disease is more advanced. Sadly, women are also more likely than men to drop out of cardiac rehabilitation programs after a heart attack.

Other Heart Conditions
Arrhythmias
Usually, the heart beats 60 to 100 times per minute with the same lapse between each beat. Arrhythmia represents an irregular rhythm. There are several types of arrhythmia which vary in degrees of dangerousness. Some are linked to underlying heart disease, others to low thyroid, iron deficiency, anemia, magnesium deficiency, and stress. Ventricular tachycardia and ventricular fibrillation are potentially fatal. In atrial fibrillation, which occurs in one percent of people over the age of 60, the heart seems to quiver instead of beating regularly because electrical impulses have been disturbed. If the underlying cause is treated, an arrhythmia will often settle down on its own.

Heart Attack Symptoms

For men and women
Episodes of angina (chest pain) that increase

Uncomfortable pressure, squeezing, tightness, fullness, or burning ache in the chest

Sweating, nausea, fainting, and dizziness

Shortness of breath

Pain or discomfort that radiates to the shoulders, arms, neck, upper back, or jaw

For women
Unusual fatigue that worsens with activity, tiredness, or depression

Chest cramping, dull chest pain, as if you have pulled a muscle from the center of your back to your chest

Heartburn, lower gastric pain, or feeling of indigestion

Paleness, profuse sweating

Overall feeling of weakness or illness

Feeling like a rubber band is constricting your throat

Sleep disturbances

Valve Disorders

With mitral stenosis, the heart's mitral valve has a narrowed opening that restricts blood flow from the left atrium into the left ventricle. Shortness of breath results when blood pressure builds up in the atrium and affects the lungs. If the valve develops a leak, blood flows backward into the heart chamber, requiring the heart to work harder and, over time, possibly resulting in heart failure. Causes include mitral valve prolapse, infectious bacteria, or a damaged heart muscle.

In aortic stenosis, a narrowed aortic valve reduces blood flow from the heart to the rest of the body. The left ventricle enlarges due to the strain, possibly resulting in angina or faintness. If left unrepaired by surgery, congestive heart failure and death may result. The aortic valve can also develop a leak, eventually causing heart failure if untended.

Heart Failure

When the heart muscle is weak, damaged, and/or abnormally thick, it becomes an inefficient pump. The result is insufficient blood flow to the body that leads to heart failure. As the body tries to compensate, symptoms include a higher heart rate, increased blood pressure, and fluid retention. As the current population living with heart disease rises, so does the incidence of heart failure. Acute heart failure occurs when the heart suddenly stops pumping efficiently. Blood backs up in the pulmonary veins, and the pressure causes the lungs to fill with fluid (pulmonary edema), creating an emergency situation.

The most common cause of heart failure is coronary artery disease, which usually occurs after one or more heart attacks and resultant high blood pressure. Other causes include valvular heart disease, inflammatory viruses and diseases, and damage caused by alcohol and drug use. Symptoms include swelling (edema) of the legs, feet, or abdomen, shortness of breath, a nighttime cough, fatigue, chest pain and pressure, weight gain, and dizziness. Keep in mind that not everyone with progressive heart failure exhibits symptoms.

The Monday Factor

Heart attacks can happen any time, yet a *British Medical Journal* study showed 20 percent more occur on Monday mornings. Similarly, a 2005 Japanese study found that blood pressure rises at the beginning of the week. If these results are not indicative of a relationship between heart health and stress, then what is? Lots of us are heading back to work after a weekend of freedom. Maybe we are thinking about a project that is due, a staff meeting we are dreading, or a temperamental boss. The result: our stress levels rise and our adrenal glands, which naturally release more adrenaline in the mornings, pump out more of this stress hormone (adrenaline is also thought to contribute to plaque rupture). Our heart rate rises and, all too often, we begin to experience one or more heart attack symptoms.

Interestingly, we now know that heart failure differs between the sexes. In men, it is usually due to systolic dysfunction, meaning that the heart is weakened, enlarged, and cannot sufficiently pump blood throughout the body. This is often referred to as a "floppy heart." Women, meanwhile, have what is described as a "stiff heart" that is associated with what is known as diastolic dysfunction, meaning that the heart's ability to relax between beats is impaired. A stiff heart muscle is small and cannot fill normally with blood. Regardless of whether your heart is floppy or stiff, heart failure is treatable and should be monitored.

The expression "An ounce of prevention is worth a pound of cure" applies to no condition better than to heart disease. By taking proactive steps to address those risk factors we can change, we can stave off or even avoid intrusive conventional medical treatment and reduce the need for medications. A multidimensional approach to heart health greatly improves our quality of life, and helps return our focus to the things that matter most in our lives.

2. Heart Disease Risks

"Keep love in your heart. A life without it is like
a sunless garden when the flowers are dead."
— Oscar Wilde

About 8 out of 10 people have at least one risk factor for heart disease, while 1 in 10 has at least three or more. The more risk factors we have, the higher the risk of developing this progressive condition. Some risk factors we are born with; others we develop — mostly from neglect or because we are just unaware. Luckily, we can reduce our risk factors through diet, lifestyle, exercise, supplements, and attention to stress and mental/emotional health.

Age

Aging inevitably puts us at higher risk of developing health issues. Our systems wear down. Heart function slows, and our arteries lose flexibility and slowly fill with plaque. About 80 percent of people 65 and older have some form of heart disease caused by a sedentary lifestyle, more stress, and higher cholesterol, to name a few contributors. People of this age group also have a greater likelihood of having high blood pressure or diabetes. Compared to men, women's overall health by the time they are diagnosed with heart disease is worse, as is the progression of the disease itself.

Although heart disease tends to show up in adulthood, younger generations are not immune to the processes that lead to this condition. Atherosclerosis can start as early as childhood. Rising rates of diabetes and obesity in kids and young adults also put them at greater risk for future health problems. A team of U.S. researchers recently did a statistical analysis to determine the potential impact between overweight adolescents and future adult heart health. They estimated that, by 2020, when the teens in the analysis turn 35, 37 percent of the males and 44 percent of the females will be obese, resulting in more heart attacks, chronic angina, and deaths by age 50. They also estimated an additional 100,000 cases of heart disease by 2035, and up to a 19 percent increase in obesity-related coronary heart disease deaths. Clearly, if only from a cardiovascular perspective, it is critically important that we promote healthy eating and fitness principles at a young age and instil in our children positive lifelong habits.

Gender

Heart disease is the leading cause of death in North America for both sexes. Until about age 40, men are more likely to suffer a heart-related event than women. After that, the tables turn and it is women who grow more at risk. After menopause, LDL levels rise, good HDL levels drop, and inflammation and C-reactive protein also increases (see Chapter 3). Female hearts are also smaller, the inner diameter of our arteries narrower, which makes the arteries more prone to blockage and damage. For women, this sizing difference could also contribute to the higher heart attack mortality rates and increased risk of complications and death after bypass surgery and angioplasty.

Low Thyroid and Hormones

Women are far more likely than men to have low thyroid function (hypothyroidism), which can worsen heart disease and its symptoms. The thyroid gland is important for metabolism, digestion, and — most importantly in matters of the heart — muscle function. When the thyroid does not produce enough thyroid hormone, the heart cannot contract and relax effectively, thus inhibiting its pumping strength. If unaddressed, dysfunction can occur during the phase of the cardiac cycle when the heart is relaxing between beats and filling with blood. In this condition, called diastolic dysfunction, the heart ventricles "stiffen," resulting in irregular blood flow and pooling. In serious cases, blood pools in the organs, mainly in the lungs, causing congestion and possible heart failure. Low thyroid function further increases C-reactive protein, a marker for inflammation. Low thyroid is also very important in cholesterol metabolism. People with severe hypothyroidism have higher elevated total and LDL cholesterol and, in 2003, the American Thyroid Association noted that even mild thyroid dysfunction can elevate blood cholesterol.

Clinical hypothyroidism is diagnosed when your thyroid-stimulating hormone (TSH) reading is higher than 5. But a TSH as low as 2 can cause low thyroid symptoms, such as fatigue, constipation, high cholesterol, weight gain, hair loss, irritability, and dry skin. If you have low thyroid function or suspect you do, have your hormone levels (re)checked.

Most cases of thyroid dysfunction go undiagnosed. Symptoms related to the cardiac-thyroid connection include:

- A slow heart beat (thyroid modulates heart beat)
- Shortness of breath, inability to exercise (caused by weakened muscles)
- High diastolic blood pressure (due to stiffer arteries)
- Swelling (edema, often a symptom of heart failure)
- High cholesterol
- Hastening of atherosclerosis

The Truth about HRT and Heart Disease

More than 100 years ago, cardiovascular disease was almost entirely a disease of men. Fifty years ago, the most popular explanations for gender-related differences in heart disease were lifestyle, including less stress for women (who were considered "happy homemakers"), and/or the fact that women did not generally smoke until World War II. Today, women who have not yet reached menopause tend to have lower rates of heart disease compared to men. Postmenopausal women in North America, on the other hand, have equal or higher rates of heart disease, with more women dying of heart attacks. Women in general also tend to have higher high-density lipoprotein cholesterol levels (the "good" cholesterol) and when women have higher good cholesterol they tend to have less heart disease than men.

We have presumed for decades that women are protected from coronary disease by a built-in factor, presumably female sex hormones. This was based on the concept that all ills in postmenopausal women have to do with declining female hormones. Several population studies suggest that a woman's universal protection against heart disease is due to estrogen. And the medical community has perpetuated this belief because coronary heart disease is less common in women before the onset of menopause; more common in women who go through a premature natural menopause; and more common in younger women who have had both ovaries removed during a hysterectomy.

Estrogen Does Not Predict Heart Disease Risk

Population-based evidence that heart disease death rates increase after menopause due to estrogen decline is actually weak. According to very thorough research published in the *Journal of Clinical Epidemiology*, there is very little evidence of a dramatic increase in heart disease due to estrogen levels in women, unlike the increase in estrogen-dependent breast cancer in postmenopausal women. Don't get us wrong. We do know that heart disease risk increases after menopause, but it has not clearly been shown to be the result of declining estrogen.

Researchers who do not support the theory that declining estrogen levels put women at risk of heart disease feel that estrogen may not be such a primary player in heart disease development as it is for breast cancer. These researchers believe that the development of heart disease may have many factors, making it much more difficult to prove estrogen's major role. Some suggest that estrogen is simply not a major factor in the development of heart disease at all. In fact, there are actually no studies, according to research published in the *British Medical Journal,* that have shown estrogen levels in the body can predict cardiovascular disease in postmenopausal women. For those of you who have read *Sexy Hormones* by Lorna Vanderhaeghe and Dr. Alvin Pettle, MD, you may already know that estrogen levels are very poorly predicted in blood, and none of the cardiovascular studies used saliva testing to get a more accurate picture of estrogen. Plus, there are many other hormones involved in heart health protection, including testosterone and progesterone.

Hormone replacement therapy (HRT) — which generally includes synthetic conjugated equine estrogens (Premarin) and synthetic progestins (remember, progestins are not progesterone) — has been available since the 1940s. Early observational studies suggested favorable effects in postmenopausal women using HRT. An increase in good cholesterol is seen in women using estrogen alone. And a deluge of other observational studies followed in an attempt to prove that HRT was the answer to postmenopausal coronary heart disease. But interestingly, along the way, most studies showed an increased risk of blood clots and heart attacks in women who had just begun HRT. Then the Women's Health Initiative study, which was designed to end the confusion once and for all about whether HRT was safe and could prevent or reduce the risk of coronary heart disease in women, was prematurely and abruptly halted in 2002 due to safety concerns. Was HRT found to be beneficial for heart disease? The answer was a resounding "No," and now a paradigm shift in the way doctors treat coronary heart disease in postmenopausal women will have to take place. Let's look at the major studies along the way.

The Coronary Drug Project

The Coronary Drug Project completed in the 1960s was the first clinical trial designed to determine whether estrogen reduced the risk of coronary events. Men with known heart disease were randomly assigned to one of five active therapies or a placebo. Two of the study medications were conjugated estrogens at a daily dose of either 2.5 or 5.0 mg; the estrogen arms were stopped early because estrogen-treated men had an increased rate of blood clots and heart attacks. After estrogen failed to protect men, no large heart-related estrogen trials were initiated in men or women for the next 23 years.

Yet, despite the absence of clinical trial data, by the middle of the

1990s, it was accepted as dogma that HRT would prevent coronary heart disease in postmenopausal women. The medical profession went so far as to consider any doctor who did not recommend estrogen therapy unethical. In the wake of this, one very important researcher, Stephen B. Hulley, believed that a clinical trial showing safety and benefit in women was essential. He obtained funding for the secondary prevention trial that came to be known as the Heart and Estrogen/ Progestin Replacement Study (HERS).

The HERS Trial

The HERS was the first large clinical trial specifically designed to evaluate whether estrogen plus progestin therapy reduced the risk of coronary events in postmenopausal women who already had coronary disease.

This study, funded by Wyeth-Ayerst, was a multiple center, randomized, double-blind, placebo-controlled trial. It included 2,763 postmenopausal women averaging 67 years of age. Each woman had an intact uterus and documented incidences of coronary heart disease. They were given a single daily tablet containing conjugated equine estrogens (0.625 mg) and medroxyprogesterone acetate (2.5 mg), or a placebo. The study lasted about four years. The HERS showed no difference in coronary heart disease outcomes between the treatment group and placebo group. Non-fatal heart attacks or coronary heart disease deaths occurred in 179 women in the hormone group and 182 women in the placebo group, meaning there was no difference. This result occurred even though LDL (the bad cholesterol) decreased and HDL (the good cholesterol) increased in the group getting HRT.

So there was no benefit. And the really scary information is that in the first year of treatment, there was a significant 52 percent increased risk of coronary heart disease events in the group using hormones. Half of the women were then followed for an additional 2.7 years and they did not show any evidence of long-term cardiovascular benefit. Stroke and peripheral artery disease also did not differ between the group getting HRT and the group getting a fake pill. In other words, HRT did not make any difference and actually increased risk of an adverse coronary event in the first year of treatment.

Great debate ensued over why the trial results did not match the belief. Researchers said the women were too old or too sick. But this was not true; the average age was 67 (the average age whereby cholesterol-lowering drugs are researched). And the women were not too sick. Most had been excluded if they had had diabetes, congestive heart failure, a recent heart attack, or vein disease. And over 75 percent of the women were compliant in the study. The one valid criticism of the study was that it was only a single trial, possibly administering the wrong hormones. But many smaller studies also showed increased risk of cardiac events. And we agree that they were prescribing the wrong hormones, including horse estrogens and synthetic progestins, which are not identical to the estrogens made by the body.

By this point, there were major studies showing an early increase in coronary death and non-fatal heart attacks in those being prescribed HRT. But the medical community still continued to prescribe hormones for the prevention and treatment of heart disease. And more women died as a result.

The PHASE Study

In this study, a team of researchers completed an un-blinded trial with 255 women who had proven heart disease. The women, averaging 66 years of age, were either given no treatment or a 17 ß-estradiol patch (2.5 mg). No synthetic progestins were given. The patch was administered alone every four days to women without a uterus or, for women with a uterus, over 14 days, followed by four patches containing 3 mg of 17 ß-estradiol and 4 mg of norethisterone. However, the study was eventually halted due to lack of benefit. After approximately 31 months, it was found that there were no differences between the group receiving hormones and the group having no treatment. But the researchers did find that, beginning in the first year, the hormone group had higher rates of all cardiovascular events except non-fatal heart attacks. Neither an increase in good cholesterol nor a decrease in bad cholesterol was observed, and this was expected due to the fact that the hormones were delivered transdermally (via the skin).

The WHI Study

The Women's Health Initiative Study (WHI) was supposed to put to rest all concerns that arose from earlier hormone studies. This randomized, double-blind, placebo-controlled clinical trial was designed to look at coronary heart disease prevention in the form of hormone therapy, diet, and calcium supplementation on disease outcomes in healthy postmenopausal women aged 50 to 79 years. In the hormone arm of the study, 16,608 women who had an intact uterus were randomly assigned to receive a single daily tablet containing conjugated equine (horse) estrogens (0.625 mg) and medroxyprogesterone acetate (2.5 mg), or a placebo. This was the same treatment given in the HERS. Another 10,739 women without a uterus were randomly assigned to placebo or conjugated equine estrogen (0.625 mg/d) without synthetic progestins. The study evaluated fatal and nonfatal heart disease and breast cancer as well as bone health.

After the first two-year follow-up, and then after one to two years, the Data and Safety Monitoring Board advised researchers that there was an early excess risk of heart attack and stroke in women assigned to both the estrogen arms. All women were sent a letter to this effect, but most women continued the treatment anyway. This is surprising, considering the risk of death. In 2002, it was found that the combined estrogen-progestin arm of this study was linked to:

- A 26 percent increase in the incidence of invasive breast cancer
- A 41 percent increase in the incidence of stroke
- A 29 percent increase in heart attacks
- Doubled rates of blood clots in legs and lungs
- A 76 percent increase in Alzheimer's dementia, according to further

evaluation of the WHI study in 2003

- Breast tissue so dense that it was challenging to detect breast cancer on a mammogram
- Increased hearing loss, according to a 2004 analysis of the data
- 37 percent reduction in the incidence of colorectal cancer, and 33 percent fewer hip fractures, which were positive notes

Even though many earlier trials showed cardiovascular risks, this trial got the attention of the media.

The PEPI Trial and Bioidentical Progesterone

The Postmenopausal Estrogen/Progestin Interventions trial was a three-year trial involving 875 women who were perimenopausal (within 10 years of menopause). This trial was not designed to study disease outcomes.

Remember, the favorable benefits of estrogen, when given alone, increased good cholesterol (HDL). And when estrogen was given with progestins, a decline in good cholesterol was discovered. In the PEPI trial, women were given either placebos, conjugated equine estrogens, conjugated equine estrogens along with synthetic progestins, either cyclical or non-cyclical, or conjugated equine estrogens and bioidentical micronized progesterone. Of all the groups, the one receiving bioidentical progesterone had superior increases in good cholesterol. This is why, in *Sexy Hormones*, it is noted that bioidentical progesterone not only opposes estrogen's negative effect on the uterine lining, it is also very important for the heart.

What Is a Woman to Do?

If you are at risk of cardiovascular disease, do not take synthetic hormones at all — not even at a low dose for the short term. Start following the program in this book to prevent and help treat any existing cardiovascular symptoms you may have. If you are suffering with menopausal symptoms and need relief, read *Sexy Hormones* and follow the safe advice for addressing menopausal symptoms.

Bioidentical Progesterone vs. Provera®

To protect the uterine lining from continuous stimulation by estrogen, most physicians prescribing standard estrogen repletion therapy (ERT) combine it with Provera®. If you ask if it is progesterone, you will probably even be told that it is — but it is not. It is medroxyprogesterone acetate, which is natural progesterone altered by the addition of a molecule to make it patentable and more orally absorbable. This molecule alters Provera's® effect on tissues other than the uterus.

Many women discontinue ERT because they do not like the way it makes them feel — irritable and often depressed. In contrast, bioidentical micronized progesterone is often called the feel-good hormone because it elevates mood and is calming. Women who have experienced mood swings and migraine headaches on Provera® notice complete resolution of these symptoms when switching to bioidentical progesterone. In addition, bioidentical progesterone was found to have the best effect on HDL cholesterol in the PEPI trial. This trial is the largest to date to include bioidentical micronized progesterone. Bioidentical progesterone can also act as a natural diuretic, in contrast to Provera®, which causes fluid retention and bloating.

There is, however, an even more compelling reason to avoid Provera®. Researchers have shown that Provera® can reverse by 50 percent the coronary-artery-dilating effect of estrogens and that bioidentical progesterone does not have this negative effect. This evidence comes from recent studies by a number of different researchers, and thus is unlikely to be disproved.

The WHI study has created a paradigm shift in the way doctors treat heart disease. No longer is it a medical sin to not prescribe hormones to women. Now we realize that caution is needed when prescribing hormones to *any* woman.

HRT — Calcium and Magnesium

The interesting relationship between HRT, cardiovascular disease, and the minerals calcium and magnesium was examined in a 2004 review published in the *Journal of the American College of Nutrition*. Magnesium researcher Dr. Mildred Seelig, MD, and her cohorts looked at research on estrogen replacement therapy (ERT) and/or hormone replacement therapy (HRT — combined synthetic estrogen and progestins). They considered small-scale studies, clinical practice, and the large-scale Women's Health Initiative (WHI) trial. While the WHI trial was halted prematurely due to increased cardiovascular complications, a few favorable findings (e.g., the lessening of hip fractures) that seemed to support estrogen use had been found. These researchers wanted to understand why. They considered these paradoxical results within the context of female nutritional mineral status and suggested that the amount of dietary calcium and magnesium consumed by most North American women (including the study participants) is an important factor in understanding these findings.

Dr. Seelig pointed out that although a high intake of calcium is routinely advised to protect against osteoporosis, high calcium — combined with low magnesium — might have contributed to the adverse cardiovascular effects noted in the WHI study in women who took HRT. These cardiovascular effects were largely due to clotting complications: heart attacks, strokes, and blood clots. Although the body's estrogen has been credited with improving the blood lipid (fat) profile, increasing nitric oxide secretion, dilating coronary arteries, as well as beneficial endothelial and anti-inflammatory effects, estrogen is also known to have a coagulant (blood-clotting) effect. Calcium, Dr. Seelig and her associates have pointed out, could have intensified it. Conversely, magnesium inhibits many steps in the clotting process and counteracts blood stickiness. Unfortunately, the typical North American's consumption of magnesium is sub-optimal.

Similarly, it was speculated that low magnesium contributed to the unfavorable mental effects found in women on estrogen in a later branch of the WHI study. Dr. Seelig and her colleagues examined how, through various mechanisms, magnesium enhances the beneficial effects of estrogen on the central nervous system. As well, they noted magnesium's ability to improve cerebral (brain) blood flow and protect against the deposition of a plaque implicated in dementia (Alzheimer's disease).

The results of Dr. Seelig's review support the supplementation of magnesium in postmenopausal women who are on ERT or HRT. This concept is not, in fact, new. As early as the 1960s, magnesium was studied in relation to oral contraceptives, also a synthetic estrogen supplement. By the 1970s, this mineral's protective anti-coagulant effect was noted as important in order to protect oral contraceptive users from the associated risks of estrogenic birth control. At the same time, we know that postmenopausal women taking synthetic estrogen excrete more magnesium via the urine and experience irregularities in internal magnesium distribution that result in lower blood levels. Studies in postmenopausal women who took synthetic estrogen or conjugated estrogen/progestins have shown that as serum (blood) estrogen and progesterone levels increase, so does calcium — but magnesium decreases. The combined effect on these hormone-induced changes is sufficient to affect heart health directly, especially if a woman is already suffering from low magnesium levels. In younger women who are not yet in menopause, magnesium's relationship to the female sex hormones is equally important to heart health. Estrogen secretion is responsible for the better utilization of magnesium in the body and higher levels of intracellular magnesium in cardiovascular tissue. As you will read further in Chapters 6 and 9, magnesium supports numerous cardiovascular functions and protects against cardiac damage. Clearly, in considering the role of hormones in relation to calcium/magnesium in the body, it is very important that all women — especially those on The Pill or ERT/HRT — ensure optimal levels of dietary magnesium.

The role of magnesium in relation to postmenopausal bone health is important as well. When estrogen production decreases in menopause, the resulting bone loss (as evidenced in research looking at hip fracture incidence and osteoporosis rates) is a concern. As previously noted, calcium is promoted as the primary mineral needed for bone health and hardness. However, calcium alone is not the answer. High calcium without accompanying magnesium poses risks to the cardiovascular system and does not support a healthy bone matrix. Dr. Seelig and her associates postulated that magnesium is the missing element when it comes to postmenopausal bone health. Although some research has indicated a beneficial (if short-term) effect of supplemental estrogen on bone health, it is estrogen and magnesium that are required for the matrix that provides bone flexibility, which is necessary for osteoporosis prevention. In animal studies, magnesium deficiency has been associated with weaker bone matrices, and diminished bone flexibility and strength. Most human studies have indicated a connection between low bone magnesium and osteoporosis. A deficiency in all-important magnesium impairs the metabolism of vitamin D (which is also needed for strong bone health), affects the functioning of hormones responsible for bone building, and interferes with calcium regulation.

Third only to cardiovascular disease and osteoporosis, cognitive loss (including dementia) is a distressing problem among postmenopausal women and, once again, magnesium plays an underappreciated role in its prevention. Studies that have looked at hormone supplementation to treat this aspect of female aging remain controversial. A later arm of the WHI study was actually halted due to safety concerns that showed an increase in mental decline among the 2,132 ERT patients; twice as many also developed dementia, compared to the 2,215 women in the placebo group. Nevertheless, it is known that the body's natural estrogen has profound brain- and mood-enhancing effects, including the modulation of neurotransmission (the relaying of electrical messages between nerves). Estrogen's positive effect on blood lipids slows atherosclerosis not just in the arteries but also in the brain;

estrogen also enhances cerebral blood flow, and protects against inflammation and degenerative breakdown. Just how does estrogen do all this? Dr. Seelig suggested that estrogen's important role in the enhancement of intracellular magnesium might be a key. Among its many beneficial mechanisms, magnesium supports healthy muscle and artery function, and thus increased blood flow to the brain. Further, this mineral's calcium-blocking ability prevents calcium uptake in the brain after brain damage, and magnesium also protects against cerebral oxidative stress and free-radical damage.

In summary, although the therapeutic value of estrogen and calcium has received the bulk of attention when it comes to postmenopausal health, magnesium's role should not continue to be overlooked. Within the cardiovascular system, magnesium protects against the blood-clotting effects of too much estrogen and/or calcium. Related to osteoporosis prevention, magnesium is essential for hormone and mineral regulation resulting in strong bone health. Through a variety of mechanisms, this mineral protects cerebral integrity and blood circulation. For all these reasons, it is imperative for women — particularly women of postmenopausal age — to obtain optimal levels of magnesium by eating a diet rich in magnesium-rich vegetables (see page 102), and by supplementing accordingly (see Chapter 9).

Family History

Although heart disease runs in families, this risk factor is not as important as most people believe. Family history of heart disease increases risk by only 25 percent. In context, this is roughly one-tenth as dangerous as smoking. So if your mother's second cousin has heart disease, you really need not worry about this particular factor. The connection has to be quite close to qualify as a risk: a mother or sister before age 65, or a father or brother before 55. And even if you have a family history of heart disease, you do not have to eat like them.

Where genetics pale, familial behavior often steps in. If your parents go heavy on meat and potatoes and drizzle them with gravy, you will likely do the same. If you cook the same meals, you will pass these habits on to your children, too. Similarly, unhealthy behaviors such as smoking, drinking too much, and dealing with stress poorly are often learned behaviors as well. So the question appears, is it genetics or the transfer of unhealthy habits that creates the increased risk of heart disease within families?

Smoking

What can be said about smoking that you have not already heard a hundred times? Smoking causes heart harm by promoting atherosclerosis, reducing good HDL cholesterol and encouraging the formation of blood clots. Smokers die from heart disease more often — almost three times more often — than they die from lung cancer. They have double the risk of heart attack compared to non-smokers.

Women who smoke and take birth control pills experience more cardiac damage. Women who take high-estrogen birth control pills and smoke have a heart attack risk more than 35 times higher than a non-smoker. While a male smoker's risk of heart attack increases three-fold over non-smokers, female smokers have up to six times the risk of heart attack compared to non-smoking women.

Let's butt out, and get our kids to butt out. The risk of heart disease drops almost immediately after quitting, and keeps shrinking. After one year, your risk will decrease by 50 percent. People who quit smoking after a heart attack or cardiac surgery reduced their risk of mortality by 36 percent, in a 2003 Cochrane review of 20 studies.

Obesity

Can you remember the last time you lugged a suitcase up the stairs, or carried heavy groceries from your car to the kitchen? Inside your chest, your heart pumped faster. You might have been winded. You might even have had to take a break. Imagine how your body would handle that extra weight packed around your middle or squeezed somewhere onto your frame. All day, every day, your heart must work harder for you to do even small tasks, like crawling out of bed or lifting a child onto your lap. Those extra pounds put added pressure on the heart muscle to keep your blood circulating, and over time they increase your risk of atherosclerosis and heart attack.

Being 20 percent higher than your ideal weight more than doubles your chance of developing heart disease. Overweight and obesity are also associated with heart disease risk factors, including high LDL cholesterol and blood pressure, and elevated triglycerides and blood sugar (glucose). The inflammation that plays a role in plaque formation in the arteries is also linked to weight. A 1999 *Journal of the American Medical Association* study reported that obese people have higher levels of C-reactive protein, a marker for inflammation. Obese men had levels of C-reactive protein five times higher than lean men, while women's levels were even higher. Obese women were also 13 times more likely to have higher C-reactive protein levels than lean women.

Obesity in North America

- An estimated 66 percent of U.S. adults are either overweight or obese

- Between 1999 and 2004, the prevalence of obesity among men increased significantly from 27.5 to 31.1 percent. There was no change in obesity among women (33.4 percent in 1999 to 33.2 percent in 2004)

- More than 17 percent of U.S. children and adolescents 2 to 19 years of age are overweight

- Twenty-three percent of adult Canadians are obese. Another 36 percent are overweight

- In 1978/79, adult obesity was 14 percent

♥ **Health Issues Related to Excess Weight**

- Type II diabetes
- Insulin resistance
- Obesity
- High blood pressure
- High cholesterol and triglycerides
- Stroke
- Osteoarthritis
- Osteoporosis
- Early death
- Accelerated aging
- Depression
- Weak immune system
- Pain and inflammation
- Extreme menopause symptoms
- Gout
- Cancer
- Kidney disease

One standard way to measure overweight and obesity is with the body mass index (BMI). One advantage of this calculation is that it considers both our weight and our height. Calculate your percentage of body fat fairly accurately by cross-matching your figures on the following chart.

BMI	19	20	21	22	23	24	25	26	27	28	29	30	31	32	33	34	35
Height	Weight (in pounds)																
4'10"	91	96	100	105	110	115	119	124	129	134	138	143	148	153	158	162	167
4'11"	94	99	104	109	114	119	124	128	133	138	143	148	153	158	163	168	173
5'	97	102	107	112	118	123	128	133	138	143	148	153	158	163	168	174	179
5'1"	100	106	111	116	122	127	132	137	143	148	153	158	164	169	174	180	185
5'2"	104	109	115	120	126	131	136	142	147	153	158	164	169	175	180	186	191
5'3"	107	113	118	124	130	135	141	146	152	158	163	169	175	180	186	191	197
5'4"	110	116	122	128	134	140	145	151	157	163	169	174	180	186	192	197	204
5'5"	114	120	126	132	138	144	150	156	162	168	174	180	186	192	198	204	210
5'6"	118	124	130	136	142	148	155	161	167	173	179	186	192	198	204	210	216
5'7"	121	127	134	140	146	153	159	166	172	178	185	191	198	204	211	217	223
5'8"	125	131	138	144	151	158	164	171	177	184	190	197	203	210	216	223	230
5'9"	128	135	142	149	155	162	169	176	182	189	196	203	209	216	223	230	236
5'10"	132	139	146	153	160	167	174	181	188	195	202	209	216	222	229	236	243
5'11"	136	143	150	157	165	172	179	186	193	200	208	215	222	229	236	243	250
6'	140	147	154	162	169	177	184	191	199	206	213	221	228	235	242	250	258
6'1"	144	151	159	166	174	182	189	197	204	212	219	227	235	242	250	257	265
6'2"	148	155	163	171	179	186	194	202	210	218	225	233	241	249	256	264	272
6'3"	152	160	168	176	184	192	200	208	216	224	232	240	248	256	264	272	279

Source: Evidence Report of Clinical Guidelines on the Identification, Evaluation, and Treatment of Overweight and Obesity in Adults, 1998. NIH/National Heart, Lung, and Blood Institute (NHLBI)

A healthy BMI reading falls between 18.5 and 24, while anything above that puts us at increased risk of heart disease. Twenty-five to 29 is overweight, while 30 or more is considered obese. If you are a trained athlete, your weight based on a measured percentage of body fat would be a better indicator of what you should weigh. A normal healthy man should not exceed 15 percent body fat, while the healthy limit for a woman is 15 to 22 percent.

Due to a few limitations with the BMI index, when considering body weight composition and associated health risks, experts often look at both BMI and our waist-to-hip ratio. Try this quick method yourself. You'll need a tape measure.

Step one: With a tape measure, measure the circumference of your waist at its narrowest (usually around the navel). Be sure to relax your abdomen or it won't be accurate.

Step two: Measure your hips at the widest point (usually around the large fleshy part of the buttocks).

Step three: Divide your waist measurement by your hip measurement.

For women, a healthy hip/ratio is considered to be less than 0.8; for men, less than 0.9. With ratios above these, risk of heart attack and stroke increases significantly in both sexes. Canadian researchers who studied 27,000 people from 52 countries reported in 2005 that men and women who had a heart attack had much higher waist-to-hip ratios than those who were heart-attack free.

Inactivity

Overweight and inactivity go together like baked potatoes and sour cream. Lack of exercise contributes to weight gain and also puts added strain on our hearts. Conversely, the positive effects of physical activity are well substantiated, and we know that even moderate activity can have heart-health effects. By improving vascular function, exercise strengthens the heart's ability to perform work. It also reduces adrenaline levels, improves muscular function, improves our blood lipid (fat) profile, and reduces the risk of fatal arrhythmias. Studies show that exercise can significantly prolong the life expectancy of patients with heart failure.

In the *British Medical Journal* in 2004, data from nine clinical trials involving more than 800 heart failure patients showed that, irrespective of the underlying causes of heart failure, all patients in the exercise treatment group lived longer and had fewer hospital admissions. Similar results were reported in the *Journal of the American College of Cardiology* in 2006. Almost 100 patients received either conventional heart failure therapy alone or in combination with a nine-month aerobic exercise regimen. The exercise group had significantly lower levels of a hormone (BNP) known to occur with worsening heart failure, and they had much improved cardiovascular function.

Apples vs. Pears — A Weighty Issue

Heart speaking, an "apple" shape, where excess weight is carried in the upper body, is more dangerous than extra weight carried below the waist — the classic "pear" figure. Abdominal fat (love handles) breaks down easier into fatty acids that raise blood triglyceride levels. It also contributes to inflammation and insulin resistance, both of which have implications for heart disease.

Above are just two of dozens of studies recognizing exercise's heart-healthy effects. It is important to note that you do not have to be an Olympic athlete to achieve a positive effect; even a brisk half-hour walk daily that induces a light sweat, combined with regular weight training, can strengthen your cardiovascular system and chip away at excess calories. If necessary, please work with a fitness trainer or join a local community center program to help guide and motivate you. Read more about Heart Health fitness in Chapter 10.

3. The Lowdown on Cholesterol and High Blood Pressure

"The heart has its reasons that reason does not know."
— Pascal

As we pointed out earlier, there are few substances as controversial as cholesterol, and no substance about which there is more confusion. We need cholesterol, yet it can also play an undesirable role in atherosclerosis. When small injuries or nicks occur in the arteries, cholesterol, which acts as an internal Band-aid, can get out of control and, with the help of other factors, clog arteries and increase our risk of heart attack and heart damage.

"Bad" LDL cholesterol contributes to heart disease. But it can be kept in line by "good" HDL cholesterol, which helps sweep LDL through the body and also helps prevent LDL from oxidizing. Oxidized LDL causes plaque formation, inflammation, and damage to neighboring cells. As if this were not enough, there are very low-density lipoproteins (VLDL) to watch out for. These extra-small bad cholesterol particles are more likely to both form arterial plaques and oxidize due to free-radical damage. People with lots of smaller LDL particles have a higher risk of heart disease than those with larger LDL particles.

About 40 percent of North Americans have higher than recommended cholesterol levels, although it is important to keep in mind that "recommendations" continue to evolve along with our understanding of the mechanisms behind heart disease. Traditionally, it was believed that your total cholesterol measure (derived by adding LDL and HDL levels together) was the best predictor of heart disease risk. It is now held that the ratio of total-to-HDL cholesterol is more accurate. For people with zero or one risk factor for developing heart disease in the next 10 years, a ratio of 6:1 is considered acceptable.

However, if you are at moderate or higher risk of developing heart disease with two or more risk factors — the category into which most people fall — maintaining a lower ratio through diet, lifestyle, supplements, and fitness is very important. Generally, the lower the ratio the better, with an ideal ratio being about 4:1. Dr. Julian Whitaker, author of *Reversing Heart Disease*, suggests a desirable total-to-HDL cholesterol ratio of less than 3:1.

Cholesterol Levels

Total Cholesterol	US (mg/dL)	Canada (mmol/L)
Ideal	<200	<5.2
High	201-239	5.2-6.1
Very High	>240	>6.2
LDL Cholesterol	US (mg/dL)	Canada (mmol/L)
Ideal	<100	<2.6
Middle Range	100-159	2.7-4.1
High	160-189	4.2-4.9
Very High	>190	>4.9/5.0
HDL Cholesterol	US (mg/dL)	Canada (mmol/L)
Low	<40	<1.0
High	>60	>1.6

The traditional cholesterol test that has been used for decades gives readings for LDL, HDL, and triglycerides, but not for newer heart disease indicators. You may require a specialized test requisitioned through your health-care provider. The newer VAP cholesterol test is very comprehensive and likely to catch on in medical testing circles although it is still relatively unused in North America. The VAP test categorizes LDL cholesterol by size, identifies HDL subclasses (some of which are more heart-protective than others), measures very low density lipoprotein (VLDL), and more. It is valuable to know your VLDL reading as another marker in your lipid (fat) profile. A "normal" VLDL reading is 5-40 mg/dL (0.1-1.0 mmol/L).

Good Cholesterol

HDL is particularly relevant to women. For women, having low HDL is ever more of a risk factor than having high "bad" LDL. Even small decreases in HDL cholesterol after menopause significantly increase the risk of heart disease. In fact, HDL cholesterol is so protective that a low amount is considered an independent risk factor for heart disease.

HDL Cholesterol Ranges

	Ideal	Increased Risk
Females	0.9-2.4 mmol/L (CAN)	<0.9 mmol/L (CAN)
to age 19	35-93 mg/dL (US)	<35 mg/dL (US)
Females 20+	>1.3 mol/L (CAN)	<1.3 mmol/L (CAN)
	>50 mg/dL (US)	<50 mg/dL (US)
	Ideal	Increased Risk
Males	0.9-1.6 mmol/L (CAN)	<0.9 mmol/L (CAN)
to age 19	35-62 mg/dL (US)	<35 mg/dL (US)
Males 20+	>1.0 mmol/L (CAN)	<1.0 mmol/L (CAN)
	>39 mg/dL (US)	<39 mg/dL (US)

Maintaining a healthy cholesterol profile is very achievable. Nine out of ten people can lower high LDL, lower VLDL, and improve HDL with dietary changes and nutritional supplements alone. Only 10 percent of people will require medication to keep levels in check. This is probably a shock to most people, considering that cholesterol-lowering statins are the number one prescribed drug in North America, and that every time official "recommended" cholesterol levels drop (as they have several times), millions more North Americans are encouraged to take pharmaceuticals to lower LDL. This raises a point to consider. How low is too low when it comes to LDL? Some research indicates that LDL may serve more of a physiological purpose than previously thought. Researchers reported in the *Canadian Medical Association Journal* last year that "LDL cholesterol levels below 2.8 mmol/L [108 mg/dL] and levels of at least 3.9 mmol/L [150.9 mg/dL] were both associated with markedly elevated risk of cancer." This study examined Type II diabetics, who are prime consumers of statin-lowering drugs due to the link between diabetes and heart disease.

Another fact pointing to the need to question current cholesterol assumptions is that many heart attack victims have "normal" cholesterol levels. This has been noted in numerous studies, including a 2009 study that looked at almost 137,000 Americans hospitalized for heart attacks between 2000 and 2006. Seventy-two percent had cholesterol levels suggesting that they were not at risk of cardiovascular disease. Many people who have heart attacks also have what is considered normal blood pressure. Clearly, another silent force is at work (see page 47 on inflammation). Cholesterol is not the universal bad guy, and although cholesterol is a factor in heart health, it is not the only factor. Rather, cholesterol should be considered as part of a complete cardiovascular health assessment.

Triglycerides

Like cholesterol, triglycerides are a blood fat. They are the most common form in the body and are manufactured in the liver. When we eat too many high-calorie, high-sugar foods (or drinks) and our body cannot burn the energy off fast enough, blood triglyceride levels shoot up and we store the triglycerides as fat. (Grab that extra roll around your middle — you're grabbing triglycerides.) Triglycerides slide through the bloodstream on the very low-density lipoprotein (VLDL) cholesterol particles that contribute to atherosclerosis and instigate free-radical damage.

Elevated triglyceride levels increase our risk of heart disease and are linked to diabetes and prediabetic syndromes such as syndrome X. Insulin resistance, which underlies all these metabolic conditions, essentially prompts the liver to produce more VLDL, which raises triglyceride levels. This fatty blood grows sluggish while its ability to carry oxygen is reduced.

Triglycerides	US (mg/dL)	Canada (mmol/L)
Desirable	<150 mg/dL	<1.7 mmol/L
Borderline high	150-199 mg/dL	1.7-2.2 mmol/L
High	200-499 mg/dL	2.3-5.6 mmol/L
Very high	500 mg/dL and above	Above 5.6 mmol/L

Fortunately, like cholesterol, triglycerides are very responsive to diet and lifestyle modifications and the nutritional supplements starting on page 165.

Lipoprotein(a) and Apolipoprotein B

Lipoprotein(a), or Lp(a), is a type of LDL cholesterol that is indicated in increased heart disease risk. One 2000 British review of 27 studies found that patients with elevated Lp(a) had a 70 percent increased risk of heart disease. Lp(a) is thought to hinder the ability to dissolve blood clots, thus increasing heart attack risk. Lp(a) also plays an inflammatory role in atherosclerosis and/or detrimentally affects the thickness and responsiveness of the arteries.

Apolipoprotein B (Apo B) is found in the VLDL and LDL particles that cart cholesterol through the blood. This small, dense protein binds with receptors on cells, promoting our uptake of cholesterol. Knowing your Apo B reading can help determine the type and/or cause of a high cholesterol reading.

Testing for Lp(a) and Apo B is less common but still available through blood work requisitioned by your doctor. If you are deemed "at risk" for cardiovascular disease, it may be covered by health-care plans. The VAP test can also detect them, although VAP testing will likely be an out-of-pocket expense.

Normal values for Lp(a) are less than 30 mg/dL in the U.S. and 0.8 mmol/L in Canada. For Apo B, the normal level is 40-125 mg/dL and a recommended 0.9 g/L respectively.

Homocysteine: Too Much of a Good Thing

To build and repair tissues and muscles, the body uses methionine, a protein. A byproduct of this repair process is the amino acid homocysteine. Unnaturally elevated levels of homocysteine in the blood damage the endothelium cells in the arteries and promote atherosclerosis. Homocysteine also stimulates abnormal growth of smooth muscle in the middle layer of the arteries, which can then thicken the wall and clog the artery in question. Homocysteine can also promote blood clots by stimulating the body's clotting mechanisms.

Elevated homocysteine triples the risk of heart attack, even after all other risk factors are accounted for. In 1997, the *Journal of the American Medical Association* reported that a high total homocysteine level represents an independent risk factor for heart disease similar to that of smoking or high blood fats (cholesterols, trigycerides). It also powerfully increases the risk associated with smoking and high blood pressure. Fortunately, the body has a built-in mechanism for dealing with too much homocysteine. We need adequate amounts of folic acid and vitamins B6 and B12 to support methylation, which converts homocysteine into harmless elements. People who are deficient in these nutrients have high homocysteine levels. We can achieve adequate levels of B vitamins through a proper diet and by taking a good multivitamin containing B vitamins, thus supporting homocysteine reduction pathways and reducing our risk of heart attack.

There is no universal "normal" or "safe" range of homocysteine, which is measured by a blood test in mmol/L. You will hear doctors say 5-15 mmol/L is standard. Most people are about 10 mmol/L, which is also the therapeutic target recommended by the American Heart Association. A typical cardiovascular risk profile ordered through a doctor sets the range at 3.0-14.0 mmol/L. Any reading above 6.3 mmol/L is associated with a steep increase in heart attack risk so the lower end of the scale is a better target to aim for.

High Iron: Dangerous

Iron is needed for hemoglobin, a protein in the red blood cells that deliver oxygen throughout the body. We also need iron for energy, muscle tone, and healthy organ function. While many people, especially vegetarians and the elderly, are at risk for iron deficiency, too much iron is an important marker of cardiovascular health. Ischemic heart disease, iron overload, and hemochromatosis (an inherited disorder where the body cannot store iron properly) are associated with high levels of ferritin, a protein in cells that stores iron so the body can use it later.

A ferritin test assesses how much iron is stored in the body. Normal serum (blood) ranges for ferritin are:

Men: 12–300 nanograms per milliliter (ng/mL)
Women: 12–150 ng/mL

Symptoms of high iron include fatigue, muscle weakness, unhealthy weight loss, and pain in the abdomen and joints. If you are diagnosed with high iron, the simplest way to reduce it is by giving blood. You can also supplement with phytic acid (1p-6), which is a natural iron chelator.

Fibrinogen: Blood Clot Indicator

Without the blood's ability to stop bleeding, even the smallest cut or scrape would be life-threatening. When a blood vessel breaks, chemical messengers and clotting factors hurry to plug the injury, then convert the liquid in the vicinity into a thicker clotty gel. One of these clotting factors is fibrinogen, produced by the liver. Although fibrinogen levels rise as we age, even in healthy people, the effects of too much fibrinogen in the body are of growing interest in the field of cardiology.

High levels of fibrinogen put us at increased risk for blood clots and, ultimately, heart attack (as most heart attacks are caused by blood clots that form in arteries clogged by atherosclerotic plaque). A blood clot can also break away and travel via the bloodstream to lodge elsewhere. Following a heart attack, excess fibrinogen is a marker for increased mortality, according to a 2005 Italian study that followed for 42 months 92 men who had suffered heart attacks. After taking into account all other factors such as age, body mass index, blood pressure, smoking, and blood lipids (fats), fibrinogen levels were the only independent predictor of death. It has also been shown to be an independent marker for overall and cardiovascular mortality in patients with end-stage kidney disease, and as a marker for the silent brain vessel lesions that increase stroke risk. A large 2005 meta-analysis in the *Journal of the American Medical Association* noted "moderately strong" associations between usual plasma fibrinogen level and the risks of coronary heart disease, stroke, and other vascular mortality.

♥ The Stress Factor in Heart Disease

Could fibrinogen be the explanation for the clear link between stress and heart disease? The results of a very interesting 2005 Belgian study suggest so. The researchers questioned whether factors such as job stress, job control and social support impacted chronic inflammation and infection in the body. They found that, in 892 Belgian men, job stress was associated with increased fibrinogen, even after considering other factors such as age, job type, body mass index, use of medications for cholesterol and blood pressure, smoking, and alcohol consumption.

Fibrinogen tests can be ordered by your doctor, or purchased online through various direct-to-consumer companies. According to the U.S. National Institutes of Health, a "normal" fibrinogen range is 200-400 milligrams per deciliter (mg/dL) of blood. The Life Extension Foundation suggests optimal fibrinogen levels are between 215-300 mg/dL. The reference ranges on a typical naturopathic cardiovascular test profile are 175-425 mg/dL. Your reading should be considered within the context of your complete cardiovascular assessment profile. It is possible to reduce elevated fibrinogen by following the recommendations in the following chapters.

C-reactive Protein: Inflammation Agent

Inflammation is your immune system's first reaction against infection or injury. When a thorn cuts through the skin on your finger, damaging tissue and allowing invaders like bacteria into your body, your immune system goes to work immediately, sending out many different types of specialized cells, each with their own action. Mast cells — specialized immune cells — release histamine, along with other immune messengers known as cytokines, to alert your body to the problem. Histamine increases blood flow to the injured area, promoting redness and swelling. Macrophages (meaning "large eating cells"), found predominantly in connective tissue and the epidermis of the skin, then enter the fray; they also secrete immune messengers, destroy the bacteria, and clean up damaged cells. Other immune cells travel to the area, intensifying the battle, and as the area is cleared, more cells arrive to begin the healing process.

The injured area often becomes hot, red, swollen, and painful. The heat is produced by the increased blood flow to the injured area. Redness occurs because the battle and repair processes are underway. And the area usually becomes swollen because of all the fluid and immune cells at the site. Pain is often the first indicator of inflammation. It makes you take notice and stop moving the affected area to prevent further injury.

Inflammation is an effective way of ensuring that invaders do not enter your body and create havoc, but when it becomes low-grade and chronic, your immune system's army stays revved up and damages healthy tissues in the crossfire. Scientists are realizing that this life-saving process, designed to ward off bacteria, viruses, and parasites, creates disease when it's left unchecked. It leads to the painful and damaging inflammation that attacks joints, organs, or arteries.

Inflammation is a major factor in heart disease. It is the suspected reason why a surprisingly high percentage of people who have had a heart attack nevertheless have normal cholesterol and blood pressure. Even in people with normal blood cholesterol, occasionally cholesterol finds its way into the lining of the arteries and is embedded there as plaque. (Those with high blood cholesterol are at greater risk of this happening.) Our immune response causes inflammation that triggers the eruption of these plaques and the formation of blood clots that silently set the stage for heart attacks.

An Infection Connection

Certain micro-organisms tend to show up in atherosclerotic plaques and promote inflammation. One of these, Chlamydia pneumoniae, is a bacterium linked to gum disease, pneumonia, bronchitis, and sinus infections. People with advanced gum disease are more likely to have heart disease, advanced atherosclerosis, and have an increased risk of stroke, compared to people with healthy gums. The common herpes simplex virus type 1 is also thought to be a possible instigator/contributor to heart disease.

Endocarditis is a heart infection caused by bacteria invading the inner lining of the heart (endocardium). The heart valves are typically involved as well; a diseased or an artificial valve can invite bacteria to lodge on the surface and nest. This can also occur during procedures in dentistry and gut examination (e.g., colonoscopy). Symptoms include a low-grade fever, fatigue, and loss of appetite and weight. Endocarditis is usually treated with antibiotics and is quite serious, with a death rate of 20 percent.

C-reactive protein (CRP) is produced by the liver during an inflammatory response. In a large-scale Harvard study involving 540 physicians, men with the highest CRP levels were three times more likely to have a heart attack and twice as likely to have had a stroke than men with the lowest levels. One year later, in 1998, a study looked at C-reactive protein in women. This inflammatory marker beat out cholesterol levels as a predictor of heart attack or stroke. "Women who developed cardiovascular events had higher baseline CRP levels than control subjects ... Those with the highest levels of CRP had a 5-fold increase in risk of any vascular event and a 7-fold increase in risk of [heart attack] or stroke." Women using hormone replacement therapy have to be aware that estrogen (Premarin was the brand used in the studies) increases inflammation in the body and elevates CRP to dangerous levels, indicating a much higher risk of heart attack and particularly strokes.

The amount of CRP in the blood is a good indicator of how much inflammation is occurring anywhere in the body, including in the arteries. Ask your physician for a high-sensitivity CRP (HS-CRP) blood test. If you have a CRP level over 3.0 mg/L, you should follow the Heart Health Diet and nutritional supplementation program to reduce CRP quickly.

Optimal:	0.5-1 mg/L
Should be monitored:	1.0-3.0 mg/L
Indicates high levels of inflammation:	>3.0 mg/L

Cardiovascular Tests that You Should Have Done

TEST	IDEAL READINGS	
	US Units	Canadian Units
Total cholesterol	<200 mg/dL	<5.2 mmol/L
LDL cholesterol	<100 mg/dL	<2.6 mmol/L
HDL cholesterol		
Men	>39 mg/dL	>1.0 mmol/L
Women	>60 mg/dL	>1.6 mmol/L
Total-to-HDL cholesterol ratio for both countries	3:1	
VLDL cholesterol	5-40 mg/dl	0.1-1.0 mmol/L
Triglycerides	<150 mg/dL	<1.7 mmol/L
Lp(a)	<30 mg/dL	<30 mg/dL
Apo B	40-125 mg/dL	0.9 g/L
Homocysteine	6.3 mmol/L	6.3 mmol/L
Ferritin		
Men	12-300 ng/mL	12-300 ng/mL
Women	12-150 ng/mL	12-150 ng/mL
Fibrinogen	215-300 mg/dL	215-300 mg/dL
C-reactive protein	<1 mg/L	<1 mg/L

High Blood Pressure (Hypertension)

Imagine trying to squeeze dishwashing liquid through a bottle head that has become caked and blocked with solidified soap. You have to press harder for any to get out, and when it does, it shoots out erratically. A similar disturbance occurs in those of us who have high blood pressure, or hypertension. With this common condition that affects one in three Americans and one in five Canadians, the heart muscle contracts too forcefully and sends blood driving through the body with excess force. Clogged arteries can create additional resistance that causes damage in the sensitive inner endothelium layer. This "wear and tear" promotes additional plaque buildup that leads to heart disease. People with high blood pressure are more than twice as likely to have a heart attack compared to people with normal blood pressure. Hypertension also strains and eventually weakens the heart, while very high blood pressure can cause blood vessels to burst in the brain, causing stroke.

Systolic vs. Diastolic

A blood pressure reading has two parts, systolic pressure (the top number) and diastolic pressure (the bottom number). The higher systolic reading represents the pressure just after your heart beats (i.e., when your heart contracts and pushes blood out into arteries). The lower diastolic reading is the pressure while your heart is at rest, refilling with blood between beats.

The ideal adult blood pressure reading is less than 120/80, measured in millimeters of mercury (mmHg). High blood pressure is considered anything higher than 140/90.

Blood Pressure	Optimal	Normal	High Normal	Hypertension
Systolic	Less than 120	Less than 130	130-139	140 or higher
Diastolic	Less than 80	Less than 85	85-89	90 or higher

A new category of high blood pressure called "prehypertension" is between 130-139/85-89 mmHg. Sixty percent of us with prehypertension will graduate to hypertension within four years unless we make heart-healthy diet, fitness, and lifestyle changes designed to bring our blood pressure back down. Even a 1 mmHg drop in diastolic blood pressure can shrink your risk for heart disease by two to three percent.

Have your blood pressure checked regularly. High blood pressure generally does not cause overt symptoms; one-fifth of Americans and two-fifths of Canadians do not know they have it. For those people who do experience symptoms, these include headache, dizziness, nausea, and blurred vision. Like heart disease, blood pressure abnormalities respond well to non-invasive, non-medicated methods of intervention.

Causes of High Blood Pressure

- Age (blood pressure can increase with age)

- A poor diet

- Magnesium deficiency

- Too much alcohol

- Lack of exercise

- Obesity

- Stress

- Another health condition, e.g., kidney disease or thyroid dysfunction (both more common in women than men)

- Pregnancy

- Birth control pills and HRT use

- Certain drugs, e.g., amphetamines (stimulants), diet pills, and some cold and allergy pills

---

4. Diabetes and Depression: Double Trouble

"If you haven't got any charity in your heart, you have the worst kind of heart trouble."

— Bob Hope

Imagine two foods on a table in front of you. The first is a hardboiled egg, the second is a white cupcake with chocolate icing. How would these foods be broken down in your body? The protein-rich egg would slowly and steadily be digested without a spike in blood glucose (sugar). The pancreas would be triggered to produce normal amounts of insulin to assist glucose uptake into cells. That cellular uptake would be equally gradual, and you would experience an even energy level until the next influx of food, hopefully an equally healthy choice.

Since glucose is the main fuel for our brain, it is important to balance our blood sugar in a way that supplies the body's demands. But, ahhh, that cupcake is tempting. And imagine what happens when you eat it. The refined flour, void of fiber and nutrients, is used by the body in the same way as pure sugar. It hits the bloodstream quickly, demanding an influx of insulin from the pancreas, which pumps out the hormone needed to shuttle glucose into cells. The cells take a huge sugar hit, resulting in a "sugar high" that leaves you buzzing. But before you know it, that quick burst of energy is gone. You are exhausted, yet you are left craving the next sugary sweet.

Steady Sugar Destruction

The cumulative effect of unhealthy food choices is destructive. If you indulge in a steady supply of high-sugar and/or high-carbohydrate processed foods, your body systems are going to become overwhelmed. Your pancreas can get overworked and will stop producing the insulin you need. Or maybe your cells become less inclined to heed insulin's call and slow the uptake of glucose, otherwise known as insulin resistance. One third of North Americans have some form of insulin resistance in which your fasting glucose level (the amount of sugar in your bloodstream after several hours of no food or drink) is higher than normal, but not high enough for a diabetes diagnosis. Over time, if you do not address this dangerous situation, your blood sugar and insulin will continue to rise and a Type II diabetes diagnosis will result.

Type I diabetes accounts for 10 percent of cases and usually begins during childhood. In Type I diabetics, the immune system has destroyed the beta cells of the pancreas that produce insulin, so daily insulin injections are required. Nine out of ten cases of diabetes are of the Type II variety, which used to be called adult-onset diabetes but is not any longer; many children and adolescents are now diagnosed with Type II diabetes due to overweight and obesity. Our pancreas and cells shout out, "No more terrible diet and lifestyle choices!" Our heart gratefully echoes the sentiment. According to the American Diabetes Association, two out of every three people with diabetes die of some form of heart or blood vessel disease. The average Type II diabetic lifespan is shortened by 10 to 15 years because of the cardiovascular side effects of diabetes.

Not Sweet for the Heart

It is misleading to focus solely on the "diabetic" effect on the heart. It would be more accurate to refer to the heart disease risks caused by all prediabetic states, including insulin resistance, in which blood glucose levels are unnaturally high. According to a 2001 *British Medical Journal* study, even elevated blood glucose is a powerful predictor of heart disease.

Excess sugar in the blood damages blood vessels by contributing to the fat deposits on their walls, which, as we know, leads to atherosclerosis, blocked arteries, and all too often, heart attacks and heart damage. Too much sugar also makes blood thicker and stickier, hindering the blood's ability to deliver nutrients and oxygen to the cells. Circulation and blood flow slows — not a good thing, considering how much energy and oxygen the heart needs to sustain its pumping effects.

When we have too much glucose in the blood, it triggers the liver to make more bad, very low density lipoproteins (VLDL) that carry triglycerides (fats) in the blood and also cause free-radical damage. Consequently, diabetes and other irregular blood sugar syndromes contribute to high triglycerides and increase bad cholesterol. At the same time, the amount of good HDL cholesterol in the body decreases. This combination of high triglycerides, high bad cholesterol, and low good cholesterol puts us at risk for heart disease. The inflammation brigade also wants in on the action. Persistent irregular sugar regulation increases fibrinogen and C-reactive protein, higher levels of which increase artery clogging and heart attack. Type II diabetics are usually found to have CRP levels four times higher than those of non-diabetics.

Metabolic Syndrome or Syndrome X

Metabolic syndrome, also known as syndrome X, insulin resistance syndrome, or Reaven's syndrome, is a cluster of factors that puts people at risk for heart disease and Type II diabetes; doubles our risk of heart attack; and multiplies our chance of developing Type II diabetes five-fold. It is estimated that more than 30 percent of North Americans have this disorder, which is typified by a combination of three or more of the following traits and medical conditions: elevated waist circumference, high blood fats and sugar, high blood pressure, and low HDL (good) cholesterol.

Sugar Speeds Aging

Yet another biochemical process related to (pre)diabetic states and heart disease — as well as premature aging — is glycation. When blood sugar binds to and chemically alters proteins and fats, damage occurs. These damaged molecules are called advanced glycation end (AGE) products and they interfere with the way cells work. They bind with collagen and make blood vessels stiff. They also promote blood clots by attracting blood platelets, encourage the oxidation of LDL cholesterol, and create low-grade inflammation that promotes atherosclerosis.

Lifestyle Is the Best Drug

If you are even 15-20 pounds overweight, you could be at risk for diabetes and heart disease. Have a glucose tolerance test to determine how quickly glucose is cleared from your blood. "Normal" blood values for the 75-gram oral glucose tolerance test that is used to check for Type II diabetes are:

Fasting: 60-100 mg/dL
1 hour: <200 mg/dL
2 hours: <140 mg/dL.

Between 140-200 mg/dL is considered impaired glucose tolerance (or prediabetes, when the body has become less sensitive to insulin and has to work harder to control blood glucose levels). This group is at increased risk for developing diabetes. Greater than 200 mg/dL is a sign of Type II diabetes.

Sometimes, blood sugar problems that generate readings too low to be "diagnosed" by traditional tests go unaddressed and cause a variety of seemingly unrelated symptoms, including anxiety, fatigue, irritability, and poor concentration. Tested or untested, everybody can benefit by working to keep blood sugars balanced and controlling the processes that create diabetes and related long-term complications such as kidney, eye, and nerve damage.

Diabetes Prevention

In one compelling study on diabetes prevention, 3,200 non-diabetics with elevated blood sugar readings were placed into three groups: one taking a placebo, one taking a common insulin drug, and one with a lifestyle-modification program including two-and-a-half hours of exercise per week. After three years, diabetes incidence was

11 cases per 100 people in the placebo group, 8 per 100 in the drug group and 5 per 100 in the lifestyle/exercise group. In other words, while drug therapy was more effective than placebo at preventing diabetes, a change in lifestyle was the most effective. Diet and exercise intervention reduced the incidence of diabetes by 58 percent. Similar findings about lifestyle and exercise's effect on diabetes prevention have since been repeated.

A recent study confirms that by taking steps to regulate blood sugar metabolism, we can also help stop heart disease in its tracks. More than 3,000 participants with impaired glucose tolerance were separated into three groups: one placebo group, one taking a common insulin drug, and one that underwent lifestyle modifications, including a calorie-restricted diet and moderate exercise. Over three years, tests were conducted to assess blood sugar changes and trends in risk factors for cardiovascular disease, including blood pressure, triglycerides, and cholesterol levels. The researchers found that as glucose tolerance status deteriorated, cardiovascular risk factors went downhill as well. Conversely, when blood sugar regulation improved, the risk factors improved. The researchers concluded that changing your lifestyle is more effective than taking an insulin drug at improving your glucose tolerance profile and cardiovascular risk.

Clearly, heart disease and diabetes (and prediabetic states) are largely diseases created by poor choices. Let's attack two killers with the power of an active lifestyle, supported by a healthy diet, targeted nutritional supplements, regular stress-reducing activities, and good mental/emotional health practices.

The Adrenal Connection

The adrenal glands are among the most important glands in the body. These small glands release the stress-response hormones that guide the body's reaction to a stressor, as well as small amounts of other hormones such as estrogen, testosterone, DHEA, cortisol, and progesterone. When the adrenal glands are functioning poorly, for example, due to the accumulated effects of internal and external stress, an impact ripples out into the area of hormone health.

Each adrenal gland sits on top of one of the kidneys and contains two parts: the adrenal medulla and the adrenal cortex. In response to triggers from the hypothalamus, the adrenal medulla secretes hormones that are involved in our genetic "flight-or-fight" response that causes that fast, short-term increase in blood sugar levels, breathing rate, cardiac output, and blood flow (more on this in Chapter 11). The adrenal cortex is responsible for the production of hormones called glucocorticoids, including cortisol. Cortisol is a hormone that is critical to blood sugar metabolism.

The secretion of hormones by the adrenal cortex in response to stress is essential to help us deal with life's stresses over the longer term. Various adrenal hormones stimulate the conversion of protein to energy, so that energy levels remain high even after the glucose released for the fight-or-flight reaction has been used up. Adrenal hormones help maintain elevated blood pressure and create changes needed to deal with stressors such as emotional shocks, infection, high workload, weather changes, environmental chemicals, or physical or emotional trauma.

Over time, particularly over a period of continual exposure to stressors, it is possible for the adrenal glands to become exhausted to the point where they are no longer able to secrete the necessary hormones. Adrenal exhaustion is a serious concern because the adrenal glands secrete both male and female sex hormones — the androgens and estrogens — and become the prime producers of estrogens and progesterone when the ovaries "retire." In today's world, most women (and people in general) have some degree of adrenal compromise. Women are generally working a full-time job, raising children, and hundreds of other demands of daily life. Poor adrenal health undermines a woman's ability to smoothly make the transitions inherent in female life. In particular, it can compromise sleep quality, which, in turn, further compromises adrenal function.

Besides overseeing female transitions, managing the stress response and its corresponding physiological effects in the body (e.g., heart rate and breathing rate), and playing a vital role in blood sugar regulation, the adrenals have another key function that is discussed in more detail in Chapter 6. The adrenals regulate sodium and water in the body, a balance that is crucial to heart health because an improper sodium-potassium ratio contributes to high blood pressure.

Many medical doctors do not recognize adrenal exhaustion unless the glands become so compromised that disorders such as Addison's disease or Cushing's syndrome occur. Until adrenal exhaustion is recognized, the person will have most likely suffered for years from symptoms of under- or over-active adrenal function. Years of chronic stress eventually cause poor adrenal function, but prior to the organ's becoming compromised, there are usually periods of overactivity that, if untreated, usually result in inadequate adrenal function.

Herbs that assist the body in adapting to stress by supporting the adrenal glands are aptly called adaptogens. Adaptogens have a normalizing effect; regardless of the condition, they help the body maintain the constant internal state necessary for health and life itself. For example, if blood pressure is high, an adaptogen will help lower it; if it is low, the same adaptogen will help normalize it. As mentioned, the adrenals must begin replacing the sex hormones produced by the ovaries during menopause. Because adaptogens support adrenal function, they can be very important to well-being during menopause. Herbs to consider for adrenal support include Siberian ginseng, rhodiola, ashwagandha, suma, and schizandra berries, all of which are effective in normalizing the stress response and improving adrenal health. For more information on these herbs and hormone health, read *Sexy Hormones* by Lorna Vanderhaeghe with Dr. Alvin Pettle, MD. Other ways to reduce stress and improve mental and emotional well-being are covered in Chapter 11.

Heart Disease Linked to Depression

No matter where we are in terms of our health — whether we are taking proactive, preventive steps; whether we have suffered a heart attack; whether we have had surgery and live with congestive heart disease — our emotions and mental state play a huge role in heart health.

Depression sufferers are four times more likely to develop heart disease. Some suggest this is because people with depressive personalities are more likely to engage in destructive habits such as smoking, drinking, and overeating, and are less likely to regularly exercise or embrace stress reduction and healing mind-body strategies. Others favor biochemical explanations because there is a definite connection between what is going on inside our hearts, and external psychosocial factors such as how we think, feel, and react to the (lack of) people around us.

Symptoms of Depression

- No interest or pleasure in things you used to enjoy
- Feeling sad or empty
- Crying easily or unexplained crying
- Feeling slowed down or feeling restless
- Feeling worthless or guilty
- Change in appetite leading to weight gain or loss
- Thinking about death or suicide
- Concentration or memory troubles
- Trouble making everyday decisions
- Problems sleeping, especially in the early morning, or wanting to sleep all the time or "hide under the covers"
- Feeling tired all the time
- Feeling numb emotionally, perhaps even to the point of not being able to cry

---

Women More At Risk

Research shows that women are more vulnerable to depression than men. About twice as many women suffer from this affliction, a statistic echoed in most countries around the world, regardless of ethnic, racial, and economic situations. A combination of uniquely feminine factors puts women more at risk. Biologically, female hormones are intricately entwined with their emotions. Menstruation, pregnancy, postpartum "baby blues," perimenopause and menopause — these are just a few specific situations in a woman's life when hormonal chemical messengers can cause major mood fluctuations. Socially and culturally, women are also under strain from the multiple roles they play (wife, mother, career woman), while a relatively lower income puts women more at risk of depression.

If you think depression is affecting you, sharing this concern with a trusted professional is important. In a 2003 National Women's Health Resource Center survey of more than 1,000 women, although the majority reported having been depressed or having known someone with depression, almost half would not discuss matters with a health-care practitioner. This is doubly and tragically ironic, considering 95 percent of them also understood that depression is treatable. As it stands, many people with depression are not adequately treated and, in women, depression is misdiagnosed 30 to 50 percent of the time.

Achy, Breaky Heart

When we are depressed, the nervous system is stimulated and puts stress on the heart. Heart rate and blood pressure increase and the risk of irregular heartbeat (arrhythmia) rises. Depression causes dysfunction of our "happy hormone" serotonin, which then encourages blood platelets to clump together, creating blood clots that can eventually clog arteries and cause heart attacks.

People with depression have more heart attacks and are more likely to die of sudden death. In one study of 2,800 heart-disease-free participants, those suffering from major depression were three times more likely to develop fatal heart disease within four years than those who were not depressed. A 2009 study in the *Journal of the American College of Cardiology* confirmed this link, evaluating 63,000 women from the long-running Nurses Health Study (1992-2004). None had heart disease signs at the study's beginning; eight percent showed signs of serious depression. The depressed women were over twice as likely to die from sudden cardiac death, frequently caused by arrhythmia. They were also slightly more likely to die from coronary heart disease than the women without depression.

Formulate Your Heart Health Plan

Not only is depression a heart disease "precursor," but people who have a cardiac event (e.g., a heart attack) or who are in recovery mode (after a surgery) are also prone to depression, which actually increases the chance of another heart attack and/or heart-disease-related fatality. Another recent study in the journal *Circulation* also suggests that depression further increases the risk of atherosclerotic progression.

After a heart attack or surgery, it is crucially important to formulate a heart health plan. Gather a supportive team comprised of health-care advisors and family, friends, club members, someone from your religious faith — whoever you need. If depression is a part of your life, or if you think you might be depressed, your team may involve a counselor or psychologist — again, someone you feel comfortable with to help guide you to better mental and emotional health.

Lifesaving Support

Social and family life keep us healthy. People with healthier support networks report better health. Single people have higher death rates than married people. Retired men who have often given up a huge portion of their lifelong identity — their work — have almost double the risk of fatal heart attack than working men. Men and women with poor social support are more likely to suffer complications during cardiovascular surgery. In early 1980s research, Hawaiian men with large social networks (family, work, church, social groups) were less likely to suffer a heart attack, angina, or other forms of heart disease. Interestingly, the stronger a man's social connections, the lesser the risk. In 2003, in a review of that evidence, National Heart Foundation of Australia researchers concluded in the *Medical Journal of Australia* that "there is strong and consistent evidence of an independent causal association between depression, social isolation and lack of quality social support and the causes and prognosis of coronary heart disease."

♥ Pets Invited

Animals are very heart-healthy. In the aftermath of a heart attack, dog owners are significantly more likely to be alive one year later, regardless of how severe the attack, according to a National Institutes of Health study involving 421 adults. In another study involving 240 married couples, those with pets had lower blood pressure and heart rates in both times of relaxation and stress, compared to non-pet owners. Owning a dog also invites more opportunities to get out there and walk, as other studies have shown. Dog owners get more exercise, resulting in other heart benefits and greater mobility.

Anger Hurts the Heart

Faced with upsetting news or an unwanted situation, which do you think is less healthy for the heart? Clenching our fists, grinding our back teeth, and lashing out verbally, or taking a calming breath, then counting to ten, maybe even walking away, and ultimately responding with more objectivity? You guessed it. The former reaction, one of anger and hostility, causes the most internal stress. Not only can it trigger an immediate heart attack or sudden cardiac death, but it also causes more long-term wear and tear on our cardiovascular system.

In times of anger and heightened emotions, numerous physical changes are activated. We tense up as if preparing for battle. Cortisol, a "stress" hormone, surges through our system. Our heartbeat speeds up and our arteries constrict, raising our blood pressure, triglycerides, and cholesterol. Simultaneously, our heart's need for oxygen to sustain these changes increases. This set of factors is why angina (chest pain) is a common symptom during bouts of anger and panic attacks. Stress, cortisol, and other hormones, meanwhile, are also getting busy elsewhere in the body while, as we discussed earlier, the hard-working adrenal glands become exhausted (for more on stress see Chapter 11).

More than 50 years ago, the propensity toward unhealthy excitable emotions and the accompanying traits of aggression, hostility, overachievement, competitiveness, and impatience was deemed Type A behavior by two cardiologists. Type As, they argued, had a higher risk of heart disease. But over time, some aspects of their theory have been rejected, others refined. Many Type A's, it turns out, do quite well in life, managing their stronger personality traits without ill health effects. It is people prone to anger, hostility, and cynicism who are especially vulnerable to heart disease. Living in this state of chronically elevated stress hormones sets the stage for high blood pressure, arterial damage, and atherosclerosis. In one Harvard study of 1,600 participants who had had a heart attack, eight percent reported being angry in the 24 hours prior to the attack. Those who also reported intense anger in the two hours prior had double the heart attack risk. In 2009, researchers did a meta-analysis of 44 studies on coronary heart disease and anger and hostility. These emotions, they concluded, impact heart disease outcomes in both healthy populations and in people with existing heart disease. In other words, whether we have heart disease or want to avoid it, learning to appropriately handle our emotions is essential.

Gone are the days when heart disease was strictly considered a physical phenomena, the mind and body disassociated from each other. Thinking on this point has come full circle in the past few decades, supported by a growing body of research. Simply put, heal our minds, heal our emotions, heal our hearts. Healthy emotional expression and positive thoughts (and reactions) are part of a strong heart-health plan. We can stop destructive patterns and replace them with beneficial alternatives.

Learn more mood-enhancing, anti-stress considerations and techniques in Chapter 12. For now, though, do yourself a favor. Put down this book. Yes, put it down and give yourself a moment to just breathe. Place your hands at your sides or over your stomach if you wish. If you are in bed, sit up and put your feet on the floor.

Close your eyes. Focus on pulling oxygen through your nose, deep into your belly. Hold it there, at the back of your spine for a count to eight, then release.

Repeat your breathing several times, while trying to clear your mind of anything but the moment. Let the stresses of the day drain away. When you are ready, let your eyes open. How do you feel? Relaxed, refreshed?

Congratulations, you have essentially just given your cardiovascular and central nervous systems a big hug of appreciation. Maybe even better, it did not cost a cent.

Anxiety — The False Heart Attack

Poor Jack Nicholson in the film *Something's Gotta Give.* You cannot help but sympathize with his character when he suffers what he thinks is a heart attack after being rejected by Diane Keaton's character, only later to be told that he had had a panic attack instead.

Heart attacks and anxiety attacks have overlapping symptoms, so it is easy to understand where the mistake is made. Both involve an increased heart rate and an irregular beat, and both are painful and uncomfortable. With a heart attack, however, the severity of pain is usually stronger and may affect other parts of the upper body besides the chest — the arms, jaw, neck, stomach (for other heart attack and gender-specific symptoms, see page 15). Heart attack victims do not tend to hyperventilate, while people having a panic attack might (unless it was the panic attack that triggered the heart attack).

Using learned techniques, such as deep breathing and relaxation exercises, panic attacks can be controlled and heart disease slowed. Anxiety sufferers may also find benefit with 5-HTP (5-hydroxytryptophan), a metabolite of the amino acid tryptophan. Proteins in the food you eat provide amino acids, including tryptophan. Tryptophan is broken down by vitamins, enzymes, and other cofactors into 5-HTP, and 5-HTP is then turned into serotonin, our "feel good" hormone. Serotonin is also the neurotransmitter that tells your brain that you are satisfied and do not need to eat more. Serotonin deficiency contributes to weight gain, depression, sleeplessness, anxiety, inflammation, and joint pain, among other symptoms.

Extracted from the herb Griffonia, 5-HTP has been researched for the treatment of depression, anxiety, and insomnia and other sleep disorders, and comes without the potential side-effects of pharmaceutical anti-depressants and sleep aids. Look for 5-HTP that is pure and enteric coated. Enteric coating ensures the 5-HTP is absorbed in the small intestine. Poor quality, non-enteric-coated 5-HTP can cause nausea when taken in optimal doses.

Recommended dosage: start with 50 mg in the morning, 50 mg mid-afternoon, and 50 mg at bedtime. You can go as high as 200 mg three times a day, but start with the lower dosage as it is often enough for aiding sleep and reducing anxiety. With 5-HTP, relief occurs within two weeks, and it can be taken long-term with no side-effects. However, if you are taking MAO inhibitors, SSRIs (Prozac, Luvox, Paxil, Effexor, Zoloft) and/or tricyclic anti-depressants (Elavil, Tofranil, Pamelor), do not take 5-HTP without discussing it with your health-care provider; 5-HTP is used to wean people off SSRIs and other anti-depressants, but this should be done under qualified guidance.

5. Heart-Smarten Up on Carbs and Fats

"The only lasting beauty is the beauty of the heart."
— Rumi

Several times a day, we have a chance to make decisions that can, quite literally, save our lives. If we choose 14-ounce steaks and French fries, skip the salad, and gorge on ice cream, we are also clogging our system with unhealthy fats and promoting "bad" LDL cholesterol buildup and atherosclerosis. We are forcing our heart (and other organs) to work harder, increasing underlying inflammation and other markers for heart disease and ... the list goes on.

What Is a Carbohydrate?

The three main components of food are protein, carbohydrates (carbs), and fats, and all are used for fuel in the body. Although protein and fats are the main sources of fuel used for repair, maintenance, and growth of all cells in the body, in our modern-day diet we tend to eat far too many carbohydrates. When carbs are present in abundance, our bodies convert them to fat.

Carbohydrates supply your body with energy. The body converts all carbohydrates, with the exception of fiber, into glucose (blood sugar). Found predominantly in plant foods and, to a lesser extent, in milk and milk products, carbohydrates are divided into two groups: complex carbohydrates, which are made up of hundreds of sugar molecules linked together, and simple carbohydrates, which are usually made up of more than three sugar molecules.

Carbohydrates are divided into two types because their different structures have a big impact on how the body uses them. Simple carbohydrates are quickly used by the body. Complex carbohydrates, also known as "good carbohydrates," require some effort on the part of the digestive system. It takes longer for complex carbohydrates to be broken down and have the glucose (and other nutrients) gradually released into the bloodstream and distributed throughout the body. Complex carbohydrates can further be categorized as high-fiber and low-fiber carbohydrates. High-fiber complex carbohydrates are the better choice.

Refining foods can change a good carbohydrate into one that is less nutritious — for example, grains are stripped of their hulls and other fibrous parts and finely ground into flours that no longer nutritionally resemble the original food. In other cases, pulp is removed from fruits to create pure juices devoid of fiber and high in fructose. As a result, these foods behave more like a simple carbohydrate, moving through the digestive system faster, with glucose hitting the bloodstream soon after consumption. When this occurs, the body has to quickly supply a high level of insulin, the hormone that acts as the body's traffic cop for blood sugar, in order to deal with the influx.

Even worse, the parts of the plant that are stripped away in the refining process are also the parts that contain most of the vitamins and minerals. Not only do these refined foods boost blood sugar, they are also almost always devoid of key building blocks that the body needs.

Simple carbohydrates are most often identified by their sweet taste. They include fructose (fruit sugar), sucrose (table sugar), and lactose (milk sugar). Products that are predominantly simple carbohydrates are fruit juices without pulp, baked goods made with white flour (such as cookies, cakes, and crackers), white pastas and breads, and any sugar-laden food (such as gooey desserts or candies). You can identify these not only by their taste but also by checking the ingredient lists on the labels. If sugars such as fructose, sucrose, or maltose are in the top five ingredients, you are holding a potentially dangerous blood-sugar booster. These foods should be avoided or limited.

Refined Carbohydrates and Mood

If you find yourself craving refined carbohydrates like baked goods or other sugar-laden sweets, you likely need to enhance your levels of serotonin, which is your happy hormone (reread about serotonin, depression and 5-HTP in Chapter 4). When you eat an abundance of refined carbohydrates, your serotonin level does go up, but it plummets just as fast because the refined carbohydrates are processed so quickly. This will make you crave more and lock into a vicious cycle of craving, sugar highs and lows, weight gain, and depression over your perceived lack of willpower.

Shortly, you will read that protein and healthy fats provide a better source for boosting your serotonin levels. If you eliminate all white pasta, white rice, white flour, and white sugar from your diet, you'll have more energy and be able to maintain a healthy weight that supports strong cardiovascular health.

Complex carbohydrates include fiber and starches, which are found in all vegetables, legumes, beans, nuts, seeds, and whole, unrefined grains; you will want to eat more of these foods. Within this category there are foods that vary in terms of how fast they cause insulin to be released into the bloodstream. Remember, too much insulin or the fast release of insulin has health consequences and is linked to premature aging as well as to the development of diabetes and obesity, both risk factors for heart disease. To avoid this, choose mostly foods below 60 on the glycemic index.

Food Glycemic Index

Avoid foods between 60 and 100

Food	Glycemic Index (GI) Rating
Glucose	100
Potato, baked	98
Carrots, cooked	92
Cornflakes	92
White rice, instant	91
Honey	74
Bread, white	72
Bagels	72
Melba toast	70
Potato, mashed	70
Bread, wheat	69
Table sugar	65
Beets	64
Raisins	61
Bran muffin	60

Eat foods rated 60 or less in moderation

Food	Glycemic Index (GI) Rating
Pita	57
Oatmeal, large cut (not instant)	55
Popcorn, air-popped	55
Buckwheat	54
Banana	53
Brown rice, cooked	50
Grapefruit juice, unsweetened	48
Bread, whole-grain pumpernickel	46
Soy milk	44
Bread, dark whole-grain rye	42
Pinto beans	42
Whole-grain pasta	41
Apples	39
Tomato juice, canned, unsweetened	38
All-bran cereal	38
Tomatoes	38
Yogurt, plain	38
Yams	37
Chickpeas	36

Skim milk	32
Strawberries	32
Real egg fettuccine	32
Kidney beans	29
Whole-grain spaghetti, protein enriched	27
Peaches	26
Cherries	24
Fructose (limit consumption: low GI but problematic)	20

Foods below 20 can be eaten freely

These non-starchy vegetables are below 20 on the glycemic index:

Arugula	Cauliflower	Kale	Rhubarb
Asparagus	Celery	Lettuces	Scallions
Avocado	Chard	Mushrooms	Seed sprouts
Broccoli	Cucumber	Purple cabbage	Zucchini
Brussels sprouts	Eggplant		

The Low-Glycemic Solution

People with heart disease, or even those with diabetes, obesity, and cancer, will find that many of their symptoms will heal quickly if they choose mostly lower glycemic foods (below 60 GI on the glycemic index). Low glycemic foods balance blood sugar, lower the body's insulin requirements, reduce body fat, reduce blood pressure, improve the immune system, promote longevity, and provide overall enhanced well-being.

Meat, poultry, fish, eggs, fats, and oils are not rated above because they have almost no carbohydrates.

Low GI = 55 or less
Medium GI = 56-69
High GI = 70 or more

The Heart Health Diet is not devoid of all carbohydrates. Instead it is based on good carbohydrates that have a lower glycemic index and do not cause a rapid rise in blood sugar, premature aging, and cellular damage that invites atherosclerosis. You will note that we have not mentioned fruit much until now. Fruit, although a complex carbohydrate, contains high amounts of naturally occurring fructose. Some fruits are low in fiber, bananas for example, so our recommendation is to eat no more than one serving of fruit a day and ensure it is a high-fiber fruit like berries. Do not drink fruit juice that is devoid of the pulp.

♥ Watch Out for Fructose

Over-consumption of high-sugar, high-carb foods and drinks is largely to blame for rising rates of obesity and diabetes. But somehow, we have been so busy avoiding "sucrose" that "fructose," which occurs naturally in fruit but can also be a highly processed sweetener and preservative from chemically altered corn syrup, has slipped by our radar undetected. Fructose is a major contributor to the obesity epidemic. High-fructose corn syrup raises blood triglycerides, VLDL cholesterol, blood sugars, and contributes to liver disease, weight gain, and a host of other degenerative health problems associated with carrying extra pounds. By avoiding foods containing fructose (even some health foods have fructose), you will cut down on not only this sugar, but also on other sweet troublemakers.

Hearts Love Fiber

There are two types of fiber: soluble and insoluble. Soluble fiber forms a gel when mixed with liquid inside the digestive system. As it does, it locks onto cholesterol, blocking its absorption. Soluble fiber also slows the release and absorption of sugars. Examples of common foods that contain soluble fiber are oats, flax seeds, citrus fruits, apples, barley, and beans. Insoluble fiber passes through the system largely intact. It pushes bulk through the digestive tract, preventing constipation and toxin buildup, and promoting regular elimination. Food sources of insoluble fiber include green beans, dark green leafy vegetables, root vegetable skins, wheat bran, whole grains, seeds, and nuts.

The average North American eats 10 grams or less of fiber daily. Yet dietary fiber is an excellent solution to heart and weight issues. In University of Kentucky studies, participants reduced their cholesterol by 13 to 19 percent by consuming three cups (750 mL) of cooked oat bran daily. That is a lot of oat bran! Since diversity of foods is best, consume other fibrous sources such as oatmeal, barley, brown rice bran, fruit, vegetables, lentils, and navy and pinto beans. In total, women need about 30 grams of fiber daily, and men, 35 grams. This is the equivalent found in seven to nine servings of vegetables. Various fibers are also sold as nutritional supplements. Whichever you choose, acclimate your digestive tract to increased fiber slowly to help avoid digestive distress. Also be sure to increase your water intake to aid elimination.

Excellent Sources of Dietary Fiber

Food	Serving Size	Fiber (g)
Split peas, cooked	1 cup	16.27
Lentils, cooked	1 cup	15.64
Black beans, cooked	1 cup	14.96
Pinto beans, cooked	1 cup	14.71
Barley, cooked	1 cup	13.60
Lima beans, cooked	1 cup	13.40
Garbanzo beans (chickpeas), cooked	1 cup	12.46
Kidney beans, cooked	1 cup	13.00
Green peas, boiled	1 cup	8.80
Oatmeal, cooked	1 cup	8.00

Fat Phobia

In the 1980s, nutritionists and cardiologists were recommending a low-fat, high-carbohydrate diet for heart disease. Many of the people who followed this plan did lose weight initially, but eventually their beneficial HDL cholesterol dropped, their triglycerides flared up, and those pounds returned. What happened? For starters, when food companies remove fats from foods, they often replace the fats with sugar. Although a food is "non-fat" or "low-fat," it might have hundreds of calories of sugars or contain fake sugars that disrupt the body's chemistry. The sugars from a high-carbohydrate lifestyle translate into insulin resistance, which predisposes us to diabetes, premature aging, heart disease, and stroke.

Plain and simple, we need fat. Yet, like carbohydrates, there are good and bad fats. Good fats not only contain healthy heart-promoting components, they also enhance overall health. Foods containing fat make you feel satisfied, and good fats are essential for brain function. Fat is also the most concentrated source of energy your body will receive. Without the right fats in your diet, your hair will fall out, your thyroid gland will not function well, depression and low mood set in, and you will crave those refined carbohydrates that cause blood sugar problems, weight gain, increased inflammation, and heart disease. Think about giving your body good fats from foods like nuts and seeds and their oils, rather than those from poor sources such as margarines, processed oils, shortenings, lards, and foods containing trans fatty acids (cancer-causing, heart-disease-promoting fats labelled as hydrogenated or partially hydrogenated). You do not fuel your car with dirty gasoline, yet every day people pollute their bodies with toxic fats that contribute to health problems.

Good fats found in some fish, nuts, and seeds, and their cold-pressed organic oils such as flaxseed, evening primrose, echium, and borage are liquid anti-inflammatories, soothing your arteries, eating away arterial plaque, and preventing clot formation.

Saturated Fats

Saturated fats are semi-solid at room temperature and are found in animal products such as red meat (beef, veal), pork, lamb, and lard, and dairy products such as milk, cheese, and butter, as well as in some processed foods. They are generally considered "bad" fats because they are associated with increased risk of heart disease, cancer, hormone problems, inflammation, and more. Many of the foods that contain saturated fats are good sources of protein. Our recommendation is to eat these foods in moderation as part of the Heart Health Diet, and to always choose sources that are organically raised and free-range.

Not all saturated fats are equal. Good saturated fats, found in butter and coconut oil, do not clog arteries, nor do they cause heart disease. Rather, they are easily digested and a good source of fuel for energy.

♥ Butter is Better

Butter, like eggs, has been unfairly vilified by heart disease experts. Butter contains a range of short- and medium-chain fatty acids, as well as monounsaturated and polyunsaturated fatty acids. Butter is preferable to margarine, a processed product, because butter contains many healthful components, including lecithin, which helps the body break down cholesterol. It is a rich source of vitamin A, which is necessary for healthy functioning of the adrenal and thyroid glands. The vitamins A and E and the mineral selenium in butter also serve as important antioxidants in protecting against free-radical damage that can destroy tissues and weaken arterial walls. The dangers associated with butter's saturated fat components have been blown out of proportion. If used in moderation (like all good things), butter is an excellent addition to the Heart Health Diet, especially if you add an essential fatty acid component like we do in the Better Butter recipe (see page 163).

The Coconut Truth

Coconut has been wrongly branded as a nutritional evil for too long. In the 1960s, data collected from research was misinterpreted, concluding that coconut oil raised levels of "bad" LDL blood cholesterol. In fact, it was the omission of essential fatty acids (EFAs) in the experimental diet that caused the observed cholesterol problems, not the inclusion of the coconut oil.

Coconut oil is a short-chain fat that is easily digested and used by the body. Subject groups studied recently in the South Pacific for their regular use of coconut oil, exhibited low incidences of coronary artery disease and low serum cholesterol levels. Little or no change is evident in serum cholesterol levels when an EFA-rich diet contains coconut oil (or butter). Coconut oil also supports healthy thyroid function. New research shows that coconut oil also enhances metabolism, aiding weight loss.

In a 2009 Brazilian study, 40 subjects involved in a randomized, double-blind, controlled clinical trial supplemented their diet daily with 30 mL (2 Tbsp) of coconut oil; followed a balanced, calorie-reduced diet; and walked 50 minutes a day for 12 weeks. They had increases in good HDL (48.7 versus 45.0), a lower LDL-to-HDL ratio (2.41 versus 3.1), and a greater reduction in waist circumference compared to subjects who followed the same diet and fitness plan but received 30 mL (2 Tbsp) daily of soybean oil instead of the coconut oil.

Coconut oil is also a rich source of medium-chain triglycerides. It is naturally saturated, so it does not need to go through hydrogenation to stabilize it. It will become harder when it is exposed to lower temperatures. Other benefits to coconut oil are that it is slightly higher in calories than most other fats and oils, and you do not need to use as much coconut oil as you would other oils when cooking or baking. Purchase virgin, cold-pressed, organic coconut oil. It is delicious.

♥ Tips for Fat-tastic Eating

- Choose coconut butter over lard and shortening
- Skip the margarine. Choose healthy oils that are cold-pressed and organic. Make Better Butter (see page 163)
- For low-heat sautéing, use extra virgin olive oil, sesame oil, or coconut butter
- For salad dressings, use unrefined oils of flaxseed, hempseed, walnut, olive, sunflower, pumpkin seed, or macadamia nut
- For baking, use butter or coconut butter
- Don't fry foods; frying promotes free radicals, which promote heart disease and other degenerative diseases. If you burn the butter in a pan or cause oil to smoke, you have created disease-promoting free radicals
- Reduce your overall consumption of animal fats

The Deadliest Fats

The fats that are so bad they are downright dangerous are trans fatty acids. They have been processed in order to stabilize them (so the foods will last longer) through a process called hydrogenation or partial hydrogenation, which changes the chemical structure of the fat, making a liquid into a solid that is more shelf-stable. The result is the development of a more poisonous form of fatty acid. Trans fats damage the cardiovascular system, promote cancer, impair immune function, and much more. Alberto Ascherio, the lead researcher on a team gathered from the Harvard School of Public Health and the Wageningen Centre for Food Sciences in the Netherlands, published a 1999 review in the *New England Journal of Medicine*. The report stated: "Coronary heart disease (CHD) kills 500,000 Americans each year. According to our estimations, if trans fats were replaced by unsaturated vegetable oils, we would expect to see at least 30,000 fewer persons die prematurely from CHD each year."

Trans fats are abundant in restaurant fried (fast) foods, baked goods, and convenience foods, including potato chips, French fries, baby biscuits, breakfast cereals, cookies, microwave popcorn, and some margarines. They are found in all fast foods that have been cooked in oils that contain trans fatty acids. Many oils in commercially produced salad dressings — except extra virgin olive oil — also contain trans fatty acids as a result of the high-heat process used to make these oils shelf-stable.

In North America, there is a push to eliminate trans fatty acids. Mandatory laws in the U.S. and Canada now require food processors to list the trans fat content on the labels of most products. As a result, many manufacturers are creating low trans fat or trans fat free versions of their products. Restaurants are also being urged to reduce the hidden trans fat content of foods. Read food labels diligently (taking into consideration the item's entire healthfulness), order with care when dining out, and eliminate all foods that contain trans fats.

Unsaturated Fats: Not Just Good but Fabulous

Unsaturated fats are liquid at room temperature and are the "good" fats. Unsaturated fats can be further classed as monounsaturated or polyunsaturated. Monounsaturated fats remain liquid at room temperature but solidify at colder temperatures. Sources of these fatty acids include olive, canola, and peanut oils. Because canola is genetically modified rape seed, it is not recommended as part of the Heart Health Diet. Canola oil is also extensively processed, exposed to bleaching and chemical solvents that create unnatural compounds. Nor do we recommend peanut oil due to its similarly heavy refining requirements.

Extra virgin olive oil is the premium oil for the heart and should be eaten every day. The olive oil extraction method involves careful cold-pressing to retain its beneficial properties. This process adheres to thousands of years of tradition. When purchasing olive oil, do not purchase those that are classified as "light;" they have been processed to remove the good fats.

Polyunsaturated fats remain liquid at room temperature, even in colder temperatures. Recommended sources of polyunsaturated fats include oils of black currant, borage, echium, flaxseed, sesame, hemp, evening primrose, and fish.

Unsaturated fats can be further classified as omega-3, omega-6, or omega-9. Omega-9s are monounsaturated and non-essential because we can make them from other fatty acids. Olive oil is a good source of naturally occurring omega-9s. Omega-3s and omega-6s are polyunsaturated and are essential because our body can't make them.

Why We Need Essential Fats

To ward off cardiovascular disease, we must obtain beneficial polyunsaturated essential fatty acids (EFAs) from food. EFAs contain their own hormones, called eicosanoids, which are the precursors to some hormones. These special hormones act as the intracellular communications control center, balancing virtually every system in the body, including, but not limited to, inflammation, blood clotting, and blood vessel dilation. EFAs fight unhealthy cholesterol levels and arterial plaque formation. In the largest study examining the effect of dietary fat on heart disease risk, more than 78,000 women were followed for 20 years. Those with the highest polyunsaturated fat consumption (7.4 percent of energy), had one-quarter the heart disease risk of women with the lowest consumption (5 percent of energy).

The most abundant EFAs in the typical diet are omega-6s. Conflicting information abounds on the benefits of omega-6 oils, mainly because of poorly designed studies that do not make a distinction between the types of omega-6 oils.

Omega-6 oils are broken down into two types: "good" omega-6 oils that contain gamma-linolenic acid (GLA) and those that do not. Those that have GLA, including black current seed, evening primrose, echium (from the borage plant family), and borage, have been shown in clinical studies to be health protective. The richest sources of GLA are evening primrose oil, echium oil, and borage oil. Hemp oil contains minimal GLA. "Bad" omega-6 oils that do not contain GLA include corn, safflower, sunflower, canola, and soy. These oils are highly refined and have been found to be disease-promoting. (Safflower and sunflower oils are available cold-pressed and organic but should still be used in moderation as they contain no GLA.)

By limiting trans fats, and by consuming more nuts, seeds, and GLA-containing omega-6 oils, you can reduce your risk of heart disease and cardiovascular-related mortality. Omega-3 polyunsaturated fatty acids are the next piece in the heart health puzzle.

Omega-3 Superstars

When it comes to cardiovascular disease, the omega-3 essential fats have become nutritional superstars. These fats, which also play a role in brain function and normal growth and development, are found in fish, algae, krill, and seed oils such as flax and echium.

Fish and fish oils started receiving mainstream support in 1996 after the American Heart Association (AHA) reported that they reduced triglycerides in the blood and inhibited the manufacture of "very bad" VLDL cholesterol, apolipoprotein B, and "bad" LDL cholesterol. Omega-3s from fish were also found to reduce blood platelet stickiness; reduce blood pressure in those with hypertension or high blood cholesterol; influence blood clotting factors; reduce atherosclerotic deposits; and reduce the inflammation precursors fibrinogen and lipoprotein(a). The Nurses Health Study, which followed more than 84,000 women for 16 years, noted that women who rarely ate fish (less than once a month) had higher risk (29 to 34 percent) of dying of coronary heart disease. And this risk dropped relative to how often the women ate fish. In another study, men who ate two fish meals a week reduced their heart attack risk by 50 percent. Other studies have noted that fish consumption protects against stroke and sudden cardiac death.

Foods Concentrated in Omega-3s

Food	Serving Size	Omega-3s (grams)
Flax seeds	0.25 cup	7.0 g
Walnuts	0.25 cup	2.3 g
Chinook salmon, baked/broiled	4.0 oz-wt	2.1 g
Echium oil	1 tsp (5 mL)	1.5 g
Scallops, baked/broiled	4.0 oz-wt	1.1 g
Halibut, baked/broiled	4.0 oz-wt	0.6 g
Shrimp, baked/broiled	4.0 oz-wt	0.4 g
Snapper, baked	4.0 oz-wt	0.4 g
Winter squash	1 cup	0.3 g
Cod, baked	4.0 oz-wt	0.3 g
Kidney beans	1 cup	1.3 g

The American Heart Association recommends eating fish twice a week. But it also acknowledges that many types of fish and seafood contain environmental contaminants, particularly mercury. The U.S. Food and Drug Administration (FDA) advises children and women who are pregnant, planning a pregnancy, or breastfeeding, to avoid eating fish with the highest likely level of mercury contamination (shark, swordfish, king mackerel, tilefish), and to eat up to 12 ounces (two average meals) per week of a variety of seafoods that are lower in mercury (canned light tuna, salmon, pollock, catfish). For everyone else, the FDA says the risk of mercury is not a concern if fish and shellfish are incorporated into a well-balanced diet, and that the nutritional benefits outweigh the risks. However, to be on the safe side, use the calculator at www.gotmercury.org to determine a weekly suggested seafood limit based on your personal weight.

Mercury Hinders the Heart

Mercury and other heavy metals are highly toxic to the neurological system. They promote free radical formation and, at the same time, hinder the body's ability to protect against free radicals. Dr. Marc Sircus, author of *Magnesium: The Ultimate Heart Medicine*, calls mercury the most potent enzyme inhibitor that exists. The heart's overall function, electrical impulse system, and contractive abilities are all severely impacted by mercury. This invasive metal is stored in the heart. Here it further affects oxidative stress, inflammation, endothelial and smooth muscle dysfunction, unhealthy blood fat and cholesterol levels, and more. One 2002 study of Finnish men found that those with the highest concentrations of mercury in their hair also had the highest rates of death from cardiovascular disease, heart failure, and stroke.

We are exposed to mercury through dental fillings, environmental contamination, vaccine ingredients (thimerosal), and fish and seafood consumption. In addition to reducing mercury exposure, we should all protect ourselves with the most powerful mercury antidote: selenium. Selenium is an overlooked star when it comes to heart protection. Not only is this mineral important for thyroid and immune function with recognized anti-cancer effects, but a deficiency in antioxidant selenium also increases atherosclerosis, and the risk of heart attack and death from coronary artery disease. And selenium counteracts mercury toxicity.

Selenium and mercury have a strong affinity for each other; they bind together in the body into an inactive, non-toxic complex that does not cross biological barriers. This renders mercury unavailable to do its damage. People who eat a lot of seafood have built-in protection when they eat high-selenium seaweed (nori) as well. Other foods that contain selenium include meat, seafood, dairy foods, whole grains, nuts (particularly Brazil nuts in the shell), red Swiss chard, turnips, garlic, and orange juice. Since selenium is unevenly distributed in the earth's crust, the amount of selenium in the soil varies around the globe, which makes our reliance on food sources difficult if not impossible to measure. Selenium levels in the body are largely dependent on the amount of the mineral in the diet. The form of selenium within the diet has an important influence on absorption. Selenomethionine is readily absorbed from the gastrointestinal tract and is significantly better absorbed and retained in the body than inorganic selenium in the form of selenite or selenate. Organic forms of selenium, such as selenomethionine, are selenium bound to methionine, an essential amino acid. Supplementing with plant-based selenomethionine (100 mcg daily), will boost your body's stores, strengthen immunity, support thyroid function, and protect against cancer.

Echium: A Premium Heart Oil

If you are concerned about impurities, PCBs, metals, and other toxic substances in fish and fish oils, but want the benefits of omega-3s, one alternative is pharmaceutical-grade fish oil supplements that have been tested to be free of heavy metals and pollutants. Some people are also looking for plant-based omega-3 sources because they are vegetarian. Others prefer not to consume fish or fish oils because they are concerned about contaminants and the environmental impact associated with fish oils from fish farming. An excellent vegetarian option for those with these concerns is echium oil from the borage plant family.

Echium oil is an exceptional source of omega-3, -6 and -9 fatty acids. Echium contains high amounts of the good omega-6 fat GLA, as well as 15-30 percent of stearidonic acid (SDA), which is readily converted to the heart-healthy eicosapentaenoic acid (EPA). Up until now, EPA has been provided mainly from fish and fish oils and, to a questionable extent, from flaxseed oil. Flax is a Heart Health oil but not for its EPA conversion. Flax contains ALA, alpha-linolenic acid, another type of omega-3 fat that has been shown to lower levels of C-reactive protein as well as reduce the risk of heart attack and stroke. According to the Flax Council of Canada, flaxseed oil provides less than 10 percent EPA conversion in a healthy person with no conversion to DHA (docosahexaenoic acid, see below) at all. Echium, on the other hand, converts up to 30 percent EPA. No other plant oil contains such high amounts of GLA, ALA, and easily provides as much EPA as echium.

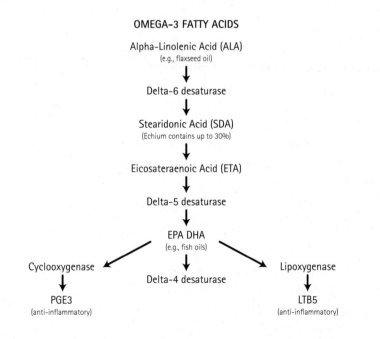

OMEGA-3 FATTY ACIDS

Alpha-Linolenic Acid (ALA)
(e.g., flaxseed oil)
↓
Delta-6 desaturase
↓
Stearidonic Acid (SDA)
(Echium contains up to 30%)
↓
Eicosateraenoic Acid (ETA)
↓
Delta-5 desaturase
↓
EPA DHA
(e.g., fish oils)
↓
Delta-4 desaturase

Cyclooxygenase
↓
PGE3
(anti-inflammatory)

Lipoxygenase
↓
LTB5
(anti-inflammatory)

In one study, EPA conversion rates were compared in 45 healthy men and women aged 18-65. They were divided into three groups who were given ALA (alpha-linolenic acid, a precursor to EPA) from flaxseed oil, SDA from echium, and EPA from fish oil. The results showed that SDA from echium oil and EPA from fish oil increased EPA in red blood cells or plasma. ALA from flaxseed oil provided no significant change in EPA levels. The researchers also found that 1 gram of SDA from echium provided 300 milligrams of EPA. A dose of 750 mg of SDA from echium increased EPA manufacture in the body up to five times that of ALA. Neither EPA from fish nor SDA from echium increased DHA levels, so DHA should be supplemented.

Echium Fights Inflammation

GLA and SDA from echium oil are powerful anti-inflammatory agents, which are beneficial in reducing the inflammation factor behind heart disease. Echium oil also lowers triglycerides, according to a 2004 study in the *American Journal of Nutritional Sciences*. Eleven subjects with high triglycerides consumed 15 grams of echium oil daily for four weeks. Eight of 11 subjects experienced decreased triglyceride levels ranging from 13 to 52 percent. In a recent animal study as well, mice who received echium oil for eight weeks experienced reductions in total triglyceride and VLDL cholesterol concentrations.

DHA (docosahexaenoic acid) is an important omega-3 fatty acid essential for the brain, nervous system, eyes, and heart. Many vegetarians, vegans, and raw food dieters are deficient in DHA unless they supplement with vegetarian algae DHA. Like fish oil, algal DHA has been shown to lower triglyceride levels and improve HDL cholesterol readings. Higher levels of DHA in the blood have been associated with reduced risks for coronary atherosclerosis progression and lowered risk of sudden cardiac death.

♥ Healthy Fat Foods and their Oils

borage	flax	pumpkin seeds
echium	fish	black current seeds
Brazil nuts	olive oil	sunflower seeds
pine nuts	hemp seeds	evening primrose
walnuts	sesame seeds	

In moderation:
butter
coconut oil

In this chapter, two key Heart Health dietary principles have been introduced:

1) Eat mostly low-glycemic carbohydrates, especially vegetables, and one serving of fruit per day.
2) Fill your fat quota with the healthy kinds of fat. Avoid margarines, processed oils, shortenings, lards, and foods containing trans fats.

Now to the next chapter, where we will look at proteins and other specific foods and nutrients that belong in the Heart Health Diet.

6. Eat the Heart-Healthy Way

"Wheresoever you go, go with all your heart."
— Confucius

If you are an Oprah fan, perhaps you caught the episode where TV personality and cardiologist Dr. Mehmet Oz discussed the revelatory results of a study looking at diet and heart disease risk factors. Eating 11 pounds of fruit, vegetables, and nuts a day is no small amount. However, after 12 days, this nutritional abundance dropped participants' cholesterol by an average 25 percent, their blood pressure dropped by 10 percent, and they lost 10 pounds each, including more than two inches around their waists. Dr. Oz says most white foods should be avoided because they are made of predominantly processed, simple carbohydrates that spike blood sugar levels and stress the cardiovascular system. To support the heart, Dr. Oz prescribes a high-protein breakfast that will curb carbohydrate cravings. He also suggests eating a small portion of protein 20 minutes before big meals to prevent overeating and mid-meal cravings. These are both sound pieces of cardiology advice.

Protein Provides Power

Our body requires 20 essential amino acids in the production of protein for cellular repair, the manufacture of hormones, immune system factors, enzymes, and tissues. Of those 20 amino acids, 12 can be made within the body; the remaining 8 must be obtained from food.

Two groups of proteins are found in the diet. Complete proteins — including meat, fish, poultry, cheese, eggs, milk, fermented soy, and whey protein powders — contain all the essential amino acids. Incomplete proteins — including grains, legumes, and leafy green vegetables — do not contain all the essential amino acids. If blood sugar is too low (hypoglycemia) from not eating enough protein, we will feel moody, lethargic, weak, and have food cravings. Protein helps keep your blood sugar stabilized, which is key to reducing body fat and avoiding the problems that too much sugar and fat cause the cardiovascular system. By eating a protein-rich breakfast, you can also increase your body's fat-burning ability by 25 percent.

♥ How Much Protein Do You Need?

Adult men	70 g
Adult women	58 g
Pregnant women	65 g
Lactating women	75 g
Girls aged 13-15	62 g
Girls aged 16-20	58 g
Boys aged 13-15	75 g
Boys aged 16-20	85 g
(Based on average weights)	

Quality protein is an important part of the Heart Health Diet. Protein from sources such as lean meats, eggs, poultry, fish, seafood, and protein powders (made of whey, pea, hemp, and/or fermented soy) provides the body with amino acid fuel.

It can be challenging to eat enough protein. If you are a sedentary woman and weigh approximately 130 pounds, you will need 45 grams of protein per day. An egg, as an example, is perfect protein and provides 6 grams. With this in mind, you can see how little protein you may be eating.

Sources of Food Protein

Dairy and Eggs	Protein (grams)
Cheddar cheese, 1 oz./28 g	7
Cottage cheese (2%), 1/2 cup	16
Egg, 1 medium, (perfect protein containing all amino acids)	6
Milk, skim, 1 cup	8
Mozzarella, part skim, 1 oz./28 g	8
Ricotta, part skim, 1/2 cup	10
Yogurt, low-fat, plain, 1 cup	12

Meat and Fish (4 oz.)	
Chicken, light meat, roasted, no skin	31
Ground beef, extra-lean, broiled	33
Sirloin steak, choice cut, trimmed, broiled	35
Tuna, canned, in water	33
Turkey breast, roasted, no skin	24

Grains	
Oatmeal, 1 cup cooked	6
Rice, brown, 1 cup cooked	5
Whole grain spaghetti, 1 cup cooked	6
Whole wheat bread, 2 slices	6

Legumes and Nuts	
Almonds, 1 oz./28 grams	6
Cashews, dry roasted, 1 oz./28 g	4
Lentils, 1/2 cup cooked	8
Peanut butter, 2 Tbsp	10
Red kidney beans, 1/2 cup canned	8
Soybeans, 1/2 cup cooked	10
Tofu, 4 oz./113 g	9

The Protein Difference

A 2006 study in the *New England Journal of Medicine* confirmed that women who follow a diet lower in carbohydrates and higher in vegetable fat and protein have a reduced risk of heart disease. This is evident in the Nurses Health Study where more than 82,000 women filled out dietary questionnaires and were followed for 20 years. Researchers noted that women with the lowest carbohydrate intake and the highest intake of vegetable proteins and fats had 30 percent lower risk of coronary heart disease compared to women who ate the most carbohydrates and fewest proteins and fats from vegetable sources. They also found that a higher glycemic (sugar) load in the body also increased risk of heart disease.

♥ Make Your Protein a Top Pick

- Eat more cold-water fish or seafood than red meat
- Choose wild fish over farmed fish
- Choose organic and free-range poultry and eggs over conventionally raised products
- Eat vegetarian proteins including legumes such as beans, chickpeas, and lentils
- Purchase nuts in the shell, and eat raw (unroasted), unsalted nuts and seeds
- Remove all visible fat from meat prior to cooking
- Choose extra-lean ground chicken, turkey, and beef. Choose leaner cuts of steak, e.g., sirloin, tenderloin, and top round
- Broiling, baking, steaming, and grilling are better than frying and deep-frying
- Overall, reduce your dairy intake

Another recent study confirmed the importance of proper protein choices. After analyzing data collected between 1995 and 2005, involving more than 500,000 men and women between the ages of 50 and 71, researchers at the National Cancer Institute found that people whose diets are high in processed and red meats are more likely to die from cancer or heart disease. Those who ate eight 4-ounce servings of red meat weekly (beef, hamburger, cold cuts, liver, sausage, pork, prepared meats in items like lasagne and pizza) had a 30 percent higher mortality than those who ate one weekly serving of meat. In heavy meat-eating men, cancer and cardiovascular-related deaths increased 22 and 27 percent, respectively. In women, the death rates of heavy meat eaters increased 20 percent for cancer and 50 percent for heart disease. This study, published in 2009 in the *Archives of Internal Medicine*, is much broader in scope than previous studies comparing the death rates of meat eaters.

The Heart Health plate should be heavy on nutritious greenery, which is an excellent source of absorbable calcium, good vegetable protein, and many other heart-protective nutrients. Your diet should be rich in EFA-rich salad dressings, low in processed and high-glycemic carbohydrates, and finished by a quality protein source about the size of your palm. Keep in mind that some people do have greater protein needs than others. If you are very active, exercise strenuously, or do heavy labor, or if you are pregnant, you will need more protein than if you are a couch potato. And since our goal is to get you up and active, be sure not to neglect your protein needs.

The Soy Story

Soybeans, soy milk, tofu, miso, and tempeh are rich protein sources also known for their cholesterol-lowering properties. Soy foods, 25 grams daily, can also lower triglycerides, raise HDL cholesterol, inhibit cholesterol oxidation, and inhibit blood clotting. The U.S. Food and Drug Administration allows soy foods with 6.25 grams or more of soy per serving to carry a heart health claim on the labels. However, not all soy is the same.

Fermented soy includes miso, tempeh, soy sauce, and fermented soy powders. Traditional Asian diets contain mainly fermented soy foods, not isolated soy protein, soy milk, or whole soybeans. Non-fermented soy foods block the production of protein-derived hormones, inhibit thyroid hormone uptake, and contain phytic acid, which can inhibit nutrient absorption. Most non-fermented soy products are also genetically modified, unless the label clearly states otherwise. In contrast, the fermentation process deactivates many of soy's detrimental effects. Fermented soy isoflavones are not as strong as conventional isoflavones, which may stimulate estrogen-receptor cells in breast tissue. However, controversy over soy's effect on abnormal cell growth lingers. For this reason, we recommend fermented soy foods only in moderation, and women with estrogen-receptor-positive breast cancer should avoid all soy products. There exists plenty of other quality sources to satisfy your protein needs.

Nattokinase for the Heart

For millennia, the Japanese have eaten natto — made from fermented soybeans — as a staple breakfast food. A component recently derived from it, nattokinase, has been labelled "the enzyme of enzymes" for its ability to dissolve certain kinds of internal congestion. Nattokinase breaks up fibrin, a protein involved in blood clotting, which makes nattokinase of great interest in cases where people have high fibrinogen levels (for a review of fibrinogen, see page 45). Nattokinase is thought to help with atherosclerosis by assisting blood clot breakup in the arteries, reducing vessel wall thickening in response to injury, and lowering elevated fibrinogen levels. If you have high fibrinogen, supplement daily with vitamin K2 MK-7 made from natto.

Calcium Can Clog Arteries

When you hear the word "calcium," you likely think of teeth and bones. Most people do because that is where calcium is supposed to lodge. However, calcium can also build up in the cardiovascular system — in the inner layer of the arteries, in the middle arterial muscle layer, and in the heart valves. Increased calcification used to be considered a symptom of aging. However, we now know that it is associated with increased arterial plaque (atherosclerosis) that builds up in response to injury, inflammation, and/or infection, and that it is an indicator that disease progression is underway. A patient with advanced coronary calcification is at increased risk of heart attack. It is important then to get enough vitamin K2, which appears to be responsible for controlling this process.

There are several forms of vitamin K. Vitamin K1 plays an important role in blood clotting, which is why people with blood clots or people who are on anti-coagulant medications (Coumadin, Warfarin) are advised to avoid foods rich in vitamin K1 such as broccoli, swiss chard, kale, and parsley. Vitamin K2 is thought more responsible for calcium deposition; it shuttles calcium out of the blood and arteries and into bones. High vitamin K2 in the body is linked to less hardening of the arteries and osteoporosis. K2 food sources include natto, liver paté, and fermented cheese. Vitamin K2 menaquinone (MK-7) from Japanese natto (fermented soy beans) in supplement form is the most absorbable and heart-healthy form of vitamin K. In a 2004 population-based study, those who supplemented with adequate amounts of vitamin K2 MK7 had a lower risk of aortic calcification and coronary heart disease than those who supplemented with vitamin K1. Participants who consumed the most vitamin K2 per day enjoyed the lowest risk of both heart attack and aortic calcification. And research has shown that vitamin K2 MK7 is better utilized than vitamin K1 and has longer-lasting effects.

Eat Like a Mediterranean

Ah, the Mediterranean — famous for its pristine beaches, magnificent scenery, holiday magic and, last but not least, its delicious food. Over the past several years, researchers have focused more and more attention on how the components of traditional Mediterranean cuisine put it at the head of the pack at both disease-prevention and aiding longevity. Not surprisingly, Mediterranean populations enjoy one of the lowest rates of heart disease in the world because their diet is based on fresh, unprocessed foods that support heart health, including:

- Abundant fruits and vegetables, which are rich in vitamins and minerals (e.g., vitamin C, E, magnesium, zinc, l-glutathione) as well as powerful plant elements (phytochemicals) known to fight cancer, and heart and eye disease
- Low-glycemic legumes (lentils, chickpeas) that convert into sugar slowly and do not require the pancreas to produce as much insulin,

thus protecting against the irregular sugar metabolism associated with (pre)diabetic states, high cholesterol, and hypertension

- Lots of root vegetables (garlic, onions) whose antioxidant properties fight free radical damage, and help lower blood pressure
- A higher consumption of seafood and fish, which contain essential fatty acids that support cardiovascular health
- Healthy fat choices, with olive oil being the primary kitchen oil
- Traditional food preparation that retains nutritive properties, e.g., foods picked riper, which allows higher nutrient development, and less frying and deep frying, which cuts down on dangerous trans fat consumption
- Lowered meat and dairy intake, i.e., less artery-damaging saturated fat and methionine, the precursor to homocysteine, high levels of which are an undesirable marker for heart disease
- More fiber-rich whole grains, fruits, and vegetables that help stabilize blood sugar and support digestive health
- Fewer processed, high-glycemic carbohydrates (e.g., white bread, white pasta) that throw off blood sugar, contribute to weight gain, encourage insulin resistance, and create fatty, sticky blood

Preserve Heart Longevity

In study after study, the traditional Mediterranean diet has justified its celebrity status. It prevents heart disease and reduces the risk of cardiac events such as heart attacks and cardiac death because the Mediterranean diet has positive effects on various risk factors, including high blood pressure, obesity, and high cholesterol. The Mediterranean diet also lowers LDL oxidation and blood fat levels. In a 2002 study involving 605 heart-attack sufferers, those on a Mediterranean diet enjoyed a 76 percent less risk of future cardiac events like heart attack, stroke, and cardiac death compared to a group eating the typical American Heart Association (AHA) diet. Fourteen cardiac events occurred in the Mediterranean group compared to 59 in the AHA diet group. Another amazing result? There were no sudden deaths in the Mediterranean diet group but eight in the other group.

Researchers looking at more than 9,400 Spanish men and women reported in 2009 that a Mediterranean-type diet also reduced blood pressure. They concluded that "a Mediterranean-type diet could contribute to the prevention of age-related changes in blood pressure." Eating like a Mediterranean also improves blood sugar regulation, helps reduce the prevalence of metabolic syndrome, and reduces inflammatory markers. A recent review of almost 200 studies and trials dated within the 60 years since diet and heart disease have been a subject of research — between 1950 and 2007 — confirms that the Mediterranean diet in its entirety is uniquely heart-healthy. After examining evidence of a potential causal relationship for various helpful and harmful factors, the researchers reported that the only dietary pattern found to be associated with reduced coronary heart disease is the Mediterranean diet.

♥ Vampires Beware

Onions and garlic, key Mediterranean foods, were the subject of a 2009 study involving 760 patients who had had a heart attack and a 682-person control group. The Italian researchers found that consuming at least one portion of onions a week reduced subsequent heart attack risk by 22 percent compared to the non-onion eaters. Likewise, garlic intake cut risk by 16 percent.

Powerful Pomegranate

For such a small fruit, pomegranate packs a powerful nutritional punch. Pomegranate is a berry; the fruit is a many-seeded berry surrounded by a juicy, fleshy outer layer. The seeds possess anti-inflammatory properties that help inhibit the enzymes responsible for inflammation and pain. Pomegranate juice has antioxidant power close to that of green tea and significantly greater than red wine. The juice has also been shown to offer protection against cardiovascular disease by reducing:

- cholesterol accumulation
- the development of atherosclerosis
- systolic blood pressure
- stress-induced myocardial ischemia in patients who have coronary heart disease
- thickening of the carotid artery

A 2004 study in *Clinical Nutrition* found that 19 patients with severe atherosclerosis of the carotid arteries who drank two ounces of pomegranate juice daily for three years had remarkable results. Ultrasound tests showed that narrowing of the arteries decreased by 35 percent on average in the pomegranate group, while the condition worsened by nearly 10 percent in the control group. The average systolic blood pressure was also significantly lowered in the group that drank pomegranate juice.

Pomegranate juice extract improves clinical gum disease, a precursor and/or indication of cardiovascular disease. In another study, it reduced the harmful products of lipid (fat) oxidation in the blood in diabetic patients without affecting insulin levels. Israeli researchers also reported in the journal *Atherosclerosis* that 50 mL of juice daily for three months slowed oxidative stress and the development of atherosclerosis in Type II diabetics. Although pomegranate juice contains sugars, it did not affect the patients' serum glucose levels.

♥ Heart Superfoods

Flaxseeds	Quinoa	Shitake
Pumpkin seeds	Pomegranate	Beans and lentils
Olives	Berries	Salmon
Walnuts	Apples	Prunes
Almonds	Spinach	

Dangerously Sugary Drinks

By now, it is hopefully clear that habitual high-sugar foods contribute to irregular sugar metabolism, insulin resistance, diabetes, and metabolic syndrome, which are all linked to heart disease. Too much sugar lowers protective HDL and raises blood pressure. Sugar orders the liver to produce triglycerides; the more you eat, the more triglyceride levels rise. Sugary foods represent extra calories that we must work harder to burn off. In addition, drinks are not exempt from a dangerous sugar influence. Regular consumption of sugary beverages increases heart disease risk. In a recent *American Journal of Clinical Nutrition* study involving 89,000 healthy women between 34 and 59, one sugar-sweetened drink daily increased the risk by 23 percent, and two or more drinks daily raised it 35 percent compared with women who consumed less than one sweetened drink per month.

Alcohol is a common source of dietary sugar. True, antioxidant-rich red wine is widely touted for heart health mainly due to its resveratrol content. Moderate consumption is thought to reduce heart disease by increasing good HDL cholesterol and by reducing blood platelet clumping and clotting. However, two or more drinks a day raise blood pressure, and given alcohol's other health effects (e.g., boosting blood sugar, disabling detoxification), only an occasional drink is part of the Heart Health Diet. If you want the antioxidant benefits of resveratrol, choose another source such as red grapes, blueberries, cranberries, or resveratrol in supplement form.

Caffeine in a Cup

When it comes to coffee, that cup o' Joe might boost energy, improve endurance, and prompt alertness, but too much can also cause headaches, indigestion, and tremors, and is linked to osteoporosis, infertility, and incontinence. Caffeine from coffee and other sources (soft drinks, medications) stimulates the nervous system and can affect heart rate. Five or more cups a day is associated with a 2.4/1.2 mmHg increase in blood pressure. Coffee can also raise levels of homocysteine, a byproduct of protein metabolism that damages arteries, and promotes atherosclerosis and blood clots.

Tea, on the other hand, contains many heart-friendly compounds — flavonoids, tannins, and catechins. In women, daily tea consumption has been found to reduce carotid plaque. A review of studies between 1990 and 2004 confirmed that three cups of black tea daily reduced risk of heart disease. Regular tea drinkers have a lower risk of heart attack; the same effect is not seen on those who drink regular and decaffeinated coffee. Green and white teas lead the tea troupe because they have more antioxidants and catechins than black tea. Be sure to choose organic black teas, as regular tea has been sprayed with anti-fungal agents. Research on these fat-fighting, blood lipid-lowering, and anti-cancer teas continues.

Herbal hibiscus tea has hearty benefits. In 2008, Tufts University researchers concluded that three cups of hibiscus tea daily for six weeks reduces systolic blood pressure. Among those patients with a systolic reading over the median of 129 mmHg, hibiscus tea consumption reduced it by 14 mmHg. Participants at or below 129 mmHg had an average drop of 7 mmHg. On a population basis, a 3 mmHg reduction would yield an 8 percent drop in stroke mortality and a 5 percent drop in heart disease mortality, highlighting the important impact that this one tea could make.

Another kind of tea that is good for heart health is ginger. Not only is ginger used by herbalists and Chinese medical doctors to treat colds, congestion, stomach upset, and digestion, but ginger, also has mild blood-thinning properties. Ginger contains gingerol, a chemical constituent that has been shown to prevent blood clotting. This herb also decreases cholesterol production. Because ginger interacts with several medications, check with your doctor if this is a concern.

The Sodium-Potassium Connection

There is much focus on the connection between sodium (salt) and elevated blood pressure. Abundant effort has also been put on salt reduction as part of blood pressure management. For instance, one landmark study, the DASH-Sodium Trial, assigned over 400 people with prehypertension and hypertension (prehypertension = 130-139/85-89 mmHg, hypertension = >140/>90) to either the standard American diet or the DASH diet. In the DASH diet group, blood pressure dropped nicely, something largely attributed to reduced sodium intake. However, salt is not the real culprit when it comes to increasing the risk of high blood pressure. The true issue is that we are not consuming enough potassium and magnesium along with sodium. While the DASH diet does reduce sodium, it also contains more vegetables that provide potassium, magnesium, and other minerals in which many people are deficient. Instead of doctors recommending to their patients to reduce salt consumption, their focus should be on encouraging patients to increase the amount of potassium and magnesium in the diet.

We need sodium to modulate muscle and nerve function, and to regulate our fluid balance and blood pressure. In northern countries like Canada and in the northern U.S., the main source of iodine in the diet comes from iodized salts. So when we tell people to avoid all salt, we get a corresponding rise in cases of low thyroid function because the thyroid needs iodine (the reason iodine was added to salt was to improve the function of the thyroid). The key to optimal heart health is that we just do not need more salt than potassium and magnesium.

Most North Americans ingest twice as much sodium compared to potassium. Some Americans consume up to 20 grams of sodium a day! But the body needs five times as much potassium as sodium. Potassium supplements would not be necessary if we simply ate more vegetables (7 to 10 half-cup servings a day to be exact). Most fruits and vegetables contain 50 times more potassium than sodium. As an example, the ratio of potassium-to-sodium in the following fruits and vegetables is:

- Apples 90:1
- Bananas 440:1
- Carrots 75:1
- Oranges 260:1
- Potatoes 110:1

Pumping Up Potassium

Like salt, potassium is influential in regulating heart function and blood pressure. It is important for cardiovascular and nerve function, for facilitating muscle energy, and for regulating the transfer of nutrients into cells. People with higher potassium-to-sodium ratios in the urine (an indicator of the potassium and sodium content of what they are eating) have far less high blood pressure than people with higher sodium-to-potassium ratios. In a Japanese study involving 59,000 men and women between 40 and 79 years of age with no history of heart disease, stroke, or cancer, a high-sodium and low-potassium intake was associated with increased risk of mortality from cardiovascular disease. Those with the highest sodium intake had a 55 percent increased risk of stroke-related death, double the risk of ischemic stroke-related death, and 42 percent increased risk of total cardiovascular disease-related mortality. Those with the highest potassium intake had a 35 percent reduced risk of heart disease-related mortality and a 27 percent reduced risk of total cardiovascular-disease mortality compared to participants with low potassium intake.

We should eat about 4,500 mg of potassium per day and avoid processed foods, which hide about three-quarters of the refined salt that the average North American eats. Plant foods, a staple of the Heart Health Diet, are an excellent source of potassium.

Secret Names for Salt

Sodium chloride (table salt)

Sodium nitrite

Sodium bicarbonate

Monosodium glutamate (MSG)

Sodium benzoate

Recommended Foods with Potassium

Food	Serving Size	Potassium (mg)
Bananas, raw	1 cup	594
Black beans, cooked	1 cup	603
Kidney beans, cooked	1 cup	704
Lentils, cooked	1 cup	720
Lima beans	1 cup	955
Potato, baked	1 potato	1081
Prunes, dried	1 cup	828
Prune juice	1 cup	707
Raisins	1 cup	1089
Spinach, cooked	1 cup	839
Swiss chard, cooked	1 cup	1016

Mighty Magnesium

Magnesium has star power and participates in numerous cardiovascular functions: increasing the heart's oxygen supply, preventing blood clots, relaxing the smooth muscles of the arteries, and slowing the blockage of blood vessels. Geographically, people who live in areas with high magnesium in the water have less cardiovascular disease and lower blood pressure. Similarly, people who consume more dietary magnesium have lower blood pressure.

We need magnesium for strong cardiovascular health, yet many calcium-channel-blocker drugs deplete the body of this crucial mineral. What an irony. Equally ironic, is that magnesium does a similar job of preventing calcium entry into cells, which allows relaxation of the arteries and improved blood flow. Besides being Nature's "calcium channel blocker," magnesium also raises good HDL cholesterol and reduces triglycerides in the blood. In a comparison of magnesium and statin (cholesterol-lowering) drugs, researchers noted similar effects on the enzymatic mechanisms associated with cholesterol development in the arteries.

Multipurpose Heart Mineral

Magnesium improves heart rates in heart failure patients, improves survival rates, clinical symptoms and quality of life in heart patients with severe congestive heart failure, reduces C-reactive protein levels (a marker of inflammation), improves exercise tolerance, exercise-induced chest pain, and quality of life in patients with coronary artery disease, and much more. Research has also shown that its relaxing effect makes magnesium valuable in cases of arrhythmia — even in life-threatening situations. One study looking at magnesium treatment immediately after heart attack found that it slashed the death rate by 75 percent and resulted in fewer complications in 96 patients. A 2005 meta-analysis of randomized, controlled trials involving magnesium use on atrial fibrillation after heart surgery found that fewer patients in the magnesium groups developed post-operative atrial fibrillation compared to the control groups (18 versus 28 percent).

Magnesium-rich foods include whole grains, legumes, and vegetables. Older adults are more at risk because magnesium absorption is affected by age. Dietary surveys reveal that most North Americans do not get even the recommended daily allowance (RDA) of magnesium, which hovers between 300 and 400 mg for teenagers and those older. RDAs are not sufficient for optimal health; we need much more than the RDA. In many cases to come, supplementing with magnesium is indicated (see page 179).

Recommended Foods with Magnesium

Food	Serving Size	Magnesium (mg)
Pumpkin seeds, raw	0.25 cup	185
Spinach, boiled	1 cup	157
Swiss chard, boiled	1 cup	151
Salmon, chinook, baked/broiled	4 oz-wt	138
Sunflower seeds, raw	0.25 cup	127
Sesame seeds	0.25 cup	126
Halibut, baked/broiled	4 oz-wt	121
Black beans, cooked	1 cup	120
Navy beans, cooked	1 cup	107
Millet, cooked	1 cup	106

By now, you are hopefully raring to get started on the Heart Health Diet. Before you embark on a new way of eating, take the heart health test on the next few pages. This will give you a starting point with which to determine what — and how much — you need to change. Then, in the next chapter, we provide plenty of tips and recipes to start you off in Heart Health style. *Bon appetit!*

7. Heart Health Personal Assessment

Circle your responses, then tally up the corresponding points and read about your heart disease risk assessment on page 108.

1. I'm ...
    Male   0
    Female   1

2. I'm ...
    Less than 30 years old   0
    30-50 years old   1
    More than 50 years old   2

3. My total cholesterol is ...
    Less than 5.2 mmol/L (200 mg/dL)   0
    5.3-6.1 mmol/L (200-239 mg/dL)   1
    Greater than 6.2 mmol/L (240 mg/dL)   2

4. My HDL cholesterol is ...
    For a woman:
    Greater than 1.3 mmol/L (50 mg/dL)   0
    Less than 1.3 mmol/L (50 mg/dL)   1

    For a man:
    Greater than 1.0 mmol/L (39 mg/dL)   0
    Less than 1.0 mmol/L (39 mg/dL)   1

5. My triglycerides are ...
    Less than 1.7 mmol/L (150 mg/dL)   0
    1.7-2.2 mmol/L (150-199 mg/dL)   1
    2.3-5.6 mmol/L (200-499 mg/dL)   2

6. My lipoprotein(a) is ...
    Less than 0.8 mmol/L (30 mg/dL)   0
    Greater than 0.8 mmol/L (30 mg/dL)   1

7. My homocysteine is ...
    Less than 6.3 mmol/L   0
    Greater than 6.3 mmol/L   1

8. My C-reactive protein is ...
    Less than 1 mg/L   0
    1-3 mg/L   1
    Greater than 3 mg/L   2

9. My blood pressure is ...
    120/80 to 130/80 mmHg   0
    130-139/85-89 mmHg   1
    140/90 or higher   2

10. I have a family history of heart disease (i.e., a mother
    or sister who has had heart disease before age 55,
    or a father or brother before 65).
    No   0
    Yes   1

11. I smoke.
    No   0
    Yes   2

12. My body mass index (BMI) is ...
    18.5 – 24   0
    25 – 29   1
    30 or higher   2

13. My body shape is that of ...
    A pear   0
    An apple   1

14. I have ...
    Diabetes   2
    Irregular blood sugar metabolism   1
    Regular blood sugar metabolism   0

15. I have ...
    Depression   2
    Previously been diagnosed with depression   1
    Never suffered from depression   0

16. I exercise _____ a week, including activities such as brisk
    walking, swimming, biking, dancing, and active gardening.
    4 or more times   0
    2-3 times   1
    0-1   2

17. I would rate my social support system as ...
    Good   0
    Fair   1
    Poor   2

18. My main sources of protein are ...
    Red meats   2
    Chicken and other poultry   1
    Seafood and fish   0

19. I eat mostly _____ daily.
    Trans fats (fried/processed foods)   2
    Saturated fats (animal fats/processed foods)   1
    Unprocessed and unsaturated fats and oils
    (of largely vegetarian origin)   0

20. My carbohydrate choices are ...
    Mostly high glycemic items   2
    Mostly medium glycemic items   1
    Mostly low glycemic items   0

21. I ...
   Eat a lot of canned foods and often add salt to my diet.   2
   Don't watch my salt intake.   1
   Watch my salt intake and try to avoid excess salt.   0

22. I drink more than 9 drinks a week (for women)
   or 14 drinks a week (for men).
   Yes   1
   No   0

23. In a typical week, I feel stressed ...
   Almost every day   2
   A few times   1
   Rarely   0

   _____

TOTAL   _____

How Did You Score?

30-39: High risk.
It's past time to start reducing your risk by making diet and lifestyle changes. We'll show you how.

20-29: Moderate/high risk.
Your heart needs help. Let's ramp up your heart-healthy efforts from medium to high speed.

10-19: Low/medium risk.
Not bad at all, but there is room for improvement.

0-9: Low risk.
Congratulations on your current heart smarts! Follow the Heart Health Program to keep you on track.

8. Heart-Healthy Recipes

"Love is space and time measured by the heart."
— Marcel Proust

Food is a miracle. It is life-sustaining and the connection between the natural world and ourselves. Let's treat our food and bodies respectfully by reconnecting with what we put in our bodies by adhering to the following eating principles. If you need to, write the following food rules on a piece of paper and post it to your fridge as a reminder at every meal.

- Eat in a calm, quiet atmosphere. Turn off the TV and phone, keeping your focus on your meal.
- Chew food thoroughly. Racing through a meal without proper chewing forces our digestive organs to work harder.
- Eat freshly cooked meals. Aim for balance, with vine-ripened fruits and vegetables for maximum nutrient content.
- Stop when you are almost full. By setting down your fork when you are 75 percent full, you avoid overeating and stressing your digestive system.
- Make the time to enjoy food. Even if it is only 20 minutes, appreciate quality mealtime, including a few minutes of relaxation afterward to aid digestion.

Getting Started

So let's get started. Before you visit the grocery store, supply list in hand, clear your cupboards and refrigerator of unhealthy foods. If you have cookies, crackers, and sweets in your pantry, you will be tempted. But if they are not in the house, you cannot eat them. Unload that freezer full of white bread and ice cream because simple sugars and carbohydrates are bad news for your hardworking cardiovascular system. When you are hungry, you will want to have the proper heart-healthy foods at your fingertips. Lean proteins and good fats and low-glycemic carbohydrates, including plenty of vegetables and unrefined whole grains, are what you are going to be stocking up on. The Heart Health rule of thumb is to choose unrefined foods that are in their natural state, and to eat organic whenever possible.

Basic Cooking Instructions
Prior to cooking, rinse grains thoroughly in cold water. Combine grain and recommended amount of water in pot/pan. Bring to a boil, then cover and simmer until ready. Use broth instead of water for different flavors.

When done, most grains should be slightly chewy. Remove from heat and gently fluff with a fork. Let sit for 5-10 minutes before serving.

Foods to avoid
- Sugary foods, soft drinks
- Artificial sweeteners
- Refined carbohydrates
- Margarine
- Unfermented soy products
- Trans-fatty acids (you'll see them listed on labels as hydrogenated or partially hydrogenated)
- Processed foods

Better choices
- All vegetables
- Fruits and their juices (no juices from concentrate)
- Organic, hormone-free meats and dairy
- Protein shakes — whey, fermented soy, pea, or rice protein powders
- Raw, unsalted nuts and seeds
- Unrefined grains
- Beans and legumes
- Unrefined EFA-rich oils such as cold-pressed flax, echium, sunflower, pumpkin seed, olive, sesame, and coconut
- Fresh herbs and sea salt

- Herbal teas (one cup of coffee per day)
- Natural sweeteners xylitol and stevia

No Fake Sweeteners

You are probably wondering whether artificial sweeteners like aspartame (NutraSweet) and sucralose are okay to use. The answer is no. Avoid them whenever possible.

Aspartame is more sinful than sugar. Aspartame is a synthetic substance made from phenylalanine, aspartic acid, and methanol (wood alcohol). Canadian laws regulate methanol, which is a potent neurotoxin, and the food supplement phenylalanine has been banned for safety reasons. Aspartame is still sold freely. Opponents of aspartame say there are links between aspartame and memory problems, seizure disorders, birth defects, headaches, and brain tumors. Although no long-term studies have proven these side-effects, there are better, natural choices available.

Sucralose is a chlorinated sucrose derivative with no long-term, human-based research conducted on its effects. A 1992 abstract published in *Science Health Abstracts* reported that large doses of sucralose shrank the thymus glands of rats by up to 40 percent. Because the thymus is so important to a healthy immune system, the Center for Science in the Public Interest, a non-profit watchdog group, requested that further studies be performed before sucralose was released in the U.S. This recommendation was ignored, and sucralose, sold under the name Splenda, is available as a sweetener in North America today. Hundreds of animal studies have been performed using sucralose, some of which show the following associated hazards:

- Enlarged liver and kidneys
- Atrophy of lymph follicles in the spleen and thymus
- Reduced growth rate
- Decreased red blood cell count

- Hyperplasia of the pelvis
- Extension of the pregnancy period
- Aborted pregnancy
- Decreased fetal body weights and placental weights
- Diarrhea

There are two safe, natural sweeteners that we recommend: stevia and xylitol. Stevia is 300 times sweeter than sugar, has no calories, and is safe for people with diabetes. Stevia leaves have been used as herbal teas by patients with diabetes in Asian countries and have been used as a sweetener in South America for centuries. In a 1993 study, no side-effects were noted in people with diabetes who used stevia for years. Two other research studies published in 1981 and 1986 found that stevia extract can actually improve blood sugar levels.

The sweet secret of stevia lies in a complex molecule called stevioside, which is a glycoside composed of glucose, sophorose, and steviol. It is this complex molecule and a number of other related compounds that account for Stevia reubaudiana's extraordinary sweetness. Stevia is available in health food stores and a growing number of drug and grocery stores in powder form for cooking and baking, and in drop and tablet form for use in coffee and tea. Xylitol, another natural sweetener, was discovered in 1891 by German chemist Emil Fischer. It occurs naturally in fruits and vegetables. Xylitol has one-third fewer calories than white sugar and reduces the development of dental cavities. Xylitol is sold as a white, crystalline powder for use as a sweetener for foods and beverages. It is also used as an ingredient in chewing gum to improve dental health.

More Heart Health Cooking Tips

To low-heat sauté, use several tablespoons of water or vegetable stock instead of oil. Cover the bottom of the pan with the ingredients you wish to sauté and slowly add more until cooked to the desired consistency. Place your large sauté pan on low heat. Add more liquid as required to prevent sticking and stir often. Sautéing in this manner will keep the temperature inside the pan at a safe level of 212°F (100°C).

Coconut oil and ghee (which is clarified butter) are the only oils that can be heated to 375°F (190°C). Certain oils, such as flaxseed, walnut, borage, or hemp, must be added at the end of cooking once the food has been removed from heat. The goal is to use as little oil as possible during the cooking process. Add oils after cooking is finished to give the satisfying flavor and texture that we crave.

With the exception of extra-virgin olive oil, supermarket oils should never be consumed, especially processed corn and canola oil. Be sure to purchase your salad dressings from the health food store or, better yet, make some of the recipes we recommend.

Never fry with any of the oils we recommend (other than coconut oil, seasme oil, or ghee), since these oils are very sensitive to heat, which will destroy their healing ingredients and make them toxic. See the chart provided below to determine cooking methods for different oils. Always add the health-giving, no-heat oils after cooking, once the pot has been removed from the heat. Fats and oils add a wonderful creamy texture and full body to foods.

- Low-heat sauté foods in water, chicken, or vegetable broth, and wine.
- Steam vegetables or fish. Boiling vegetables leaches the important phytonutrients into the water, which is then tossed down the drain.
- Poach or simmer foods, especially fish.
- Soups and stews are a safe cooking method as foods are cooked over low heat.
- Low-heat oven roasting up to 250°F (120°C) is excellent for garlic, chicken, meats, fish, and vegetables.
- When baking breads and muffins at temperatures around 325°F (165°C), the moisture keeps the inside temperature under 212°F (100°C).
- For full flavor of nut oils, add after cooking.

The best addition to any kitchen is a food processor. Choose a heavy-duty appliance that has several blades and attachments. It is invaluable when preparing vegetables, spreads, desserts, salad dressings, and much more. A food processor is used in the preparation of several recipes; it is not a requirement, just a time-saving process. If you do not own a food processor, then a good knife or a blender, coffee grinder, or hand-held blender may provide similar results.

Some of the recipes recommend certified organic, finely ground flax meal. It can be added to any of your favorite baking recipes. Just substitute the fibrous ingredients, i.e., ¼ cup (60 mL) of wheat germ can be replaced with ¼ cup (60 mL) of ground flax. We recommend that you not add more than ½ cup (125 mL) of flax to your baking recipes or the result may be a muffin, bread, or pastry that is just too heavy. To grind flax, pulse flax seeds in a coffee grinder for a few seconds. If possible, reserve a small coffee grinder expressly for this purpose.

♥ Other Healthful Advice

Do you have gas or feel bloated? Do you belch or have a big belly? Plant-based enzymes aid the digestive system. Look for a well-rounded formula in your local natural health food store.

Lactic acid in natural yogurt and sauerkraut helps enzyme production. Countries where these foods are consumed regularly (such as Russia, Bulgaria, and Romania) have lower cancer rates per capita and have the highest number of centenarians.

Tomatoes are rich in the phytonutrient lycopene, a powerful cancer-protective agent. Tomatoes should be eaten with oil to increase the absorption of lycopene.

Jalapeño and cayenne peppers contain capsicum, which is a powerful antioxidant.

Several different seed and nut oils are recommended in the following recipes. Their essential fatty acid content is important as well, as this determines the temperatures they can withstand in cooking. Each oil is chosen not only for its culinary delights but also for its essential fatty acid (EFA) content and ability to be heated (or not). Purchase organic, cold-pressed nut and seed oils.

Essesntial Fatty Acid Profiles of Different Oils

Oil	Omega-6	Omega-9	Other	
Coconut	–	7%	Saturated fat	91%
Flaxseed	15%	21%	Omega-3	54%
Echium	26-33%		Omega-3	45-60%
Hazelnut	14%	77%		
Olive	15%	63%		
Pistachio	30%	54%		
Pumpkin	55%	25%		
Safflower	78%	12%		
Sesame	45%	40%		
Sunflower	71%	16%		
Hi-oleic sunflower	15%	75%		

Temperature Chart

No Heat (120°F/49°C) Superpoly-unsaturates (condiments, salad dressings)	Low Heat (212°F/100°C) Polyunsaturates (sauces, baking)	Medium Heat (325°F/165°C) Monounsaturates (light sautéing) For optimal flavor add after cooking	High Heat (375°F/190°C) Saturates (high-heat sautéing)
Flaxseed oil	Safflower oil	Almond oil	Coconut oil
Echium Oil	Sunflower oil	Hazelnut oil	
Omega Essential Balance oil	Pumpkin oil	Olive oil	Ghee (clarified butter used in Indian cooking methods)
Udo's Choice oil		Pistachio oil	
Borage oil		Sesame oil	
Walnut oil			
Hemp seed oil			

Healthier Whole Grain Cooking Chart

Grain (1 cup)	Water (in cups)	Approx. Time (minutes)
Amaranth	2 1/2-3	20-25
Barley		
- brown	3-4	55
- pearl	1-2	40
Buckwheat, raw	3	15-20
Millet	3-4	25
Oats, whole	3-4	50-55
Quinoa*	2	20
Rice		
- brown	2	40-45
- brown basmati	2	40-45
- wild	3	55-60
Wheat		
- bulgur	2	15-20
- whole berries**	3-4	60

* Prior to cooking, rinse with water through strainer to remove bitterness.

** Whole wheat berries should be soaked overnight (8 hours) in water in a covered bowl.

Recipes

Breakfast

Granola Crunch

Ingredients
4 cups (1 L) rolled oats
1 cup (250 mL) rye
1 cup (250 mL) wheat germ
1/2 cup (125 mL) pumpkin seeds
1/2 cup (125 mL) almonds, chopped
1/2 cup (125 mL) almond butter (optional)
1/4 cup (60 mL) organic maple syrup,
     or half and half (1/8 cup; 30 mL) organic blackstrap molasses
2 Tbsp (45 mL) water
3/4-1 cup (175-250 mL) dried fruit (chopped if necessary),
     e.g., apricots, dates, raisins, cranberries, soft goji berries

Instructions
Preheat oven to 275°F(140°C). In a baking/roasting pan, add and mix oats, rye, wheat germ, pumpkin seeds, and almonds. In another bowl, using a fork, mix almond butter, syrup (and blackstrap molasses) and water. Drizzle over panned ingredients and mix.

Cover and roast for 50-60 minutes, stirring occasionally. Allow to cool, then mix in dried fruits of your choice and store in refrigerator.

Serve as desired with milk substitute (almond, brown rice). Makes about 8 cups (2 kg).

We love granola because it doubles as a great dry energy food. Take a snack bag with you when you are hiking or on outdoor summer strolls.

Protein-packed Fruit Pudding

Ingredients
1 cup (250 mL) plain yogurt
2 Tbsp (30 mL) flax meal
1/4 cup (60 mL) granola
1 Tbsp (15 mL) flaxseed oil or EFA-oil blend
1-2 scoops protein powder
Fruit of your choice (bananas, strawberries, mango, blueberries, and papaya are excellent)

Instructions
Mix all ingredients. Chill before serving, and enjoy. Makes 1 serving.

Apple Oatmeal

Ingredients
1 cup (250 mL) old-fashioned oats (thick cut are best)
1 cup (250 mL) water
1 cup (250 mL) apple juice
3 medium-size apples, grated
1 handful raisins, rinsed (optional)
Dash cinnamon
3 Tbsp (45 mL) flaxseed oil or essential oil blend
2 Tbsp (30 mL) ground flax meal

Instructions
Place first six ingredients in a heavy saucepan. Cover and cook over low heat for 20 minutes. Stir occasionally. Remove from heat and stir in oil. Spoon oatmeal into individual serving dishes and sprinkle with ground flax meal. Makes 2 servings.

Mom's Best Rice Pudding

Ingredients
3 cups (750 mL) cooked brown rice
6 eggs, well beaten
1 1/2 cup (375 mL) milk or milk substitute
1/2 cup (125 mL) maple syrup
1 tsp (5 mL) vanilla
1 tsp (5 mL) cinnamon
1 apple, grated (optional)
1/4 cup (60 mL) flax meal
2 Tbsp (30 mL) flaxseed oil
1 cup (250 mL) yogurt (optional)

Instructions
Mix together first six ingredients (and grated apple if you are using it) and pour into a buttered casserole dish. Bake in a preheated 350°F (180°C) oven for 30-40 minutes or until firm. The pudding should be thick, not runny. Once cooled, stir in flax, oil, and yogurt (if desired).

This can be served hot or cold for breakfast. Top with applesauce for a sweet treat. Makes 4 servings.

Flax Pudding

Ingredients
6 Tbsp (90 mL) flaxseeds
2 cups (500 mL) milk or milk alternative
2 Tbsp (30 mL) ground hazelnuts, almonds, or pistachios
1 large banana, mashed
Juice of one orange
1 Tbsp honey (optional)
1 apple, peeled, cored, and grated

Instructions
Pulse the flaxseeds in a coffee grinder for a few seconds. Bring milk to a boil in a double-boiler and stir in ground flaxseeds with a whisk to prevent lumps (add all of the ground flaxseed at once); boil for 30 seconds, remove from heat, and pour into a bowl. Let cool. It will have the consistency of pudding. Mix ground nuts, banana, orange juice, and honey, into the flax pudding mixture. Gently mix in grated apple and spoon into parfait dishes layered alternatively with fresh fruit. Top with a strawberry for garnish. Makes 4 servings.

This recipe is a great one for slipping children (or husbands) those beneficial essential fatty acids without them knowing it.

Applesauce Surprise

Ingredients
1 cup (250 mL) organic applesauce
Dash cinnamon
2 Tbsp (30 mL) flax meal
1/2 cup (125 mL) plain or vanilla yogurt

Instructions
To make fresh flax meal, pulse the same amount of flax seeds in a coffee grinder for a few seconds.

Mix all ingredients together and serve immediately. Makes 1-2 servings.

Rice Pancakes

Ingredients
1 3/4 cups (425 mL) brown rice flour
1/4 cup (60 mL) tapioca or arrowroot starch
1-2 Tbsp (15-30 mL) liquid honey
2 cups (500 mL) almond, hemp, or brown rice milk
3 Tbsp (45 mL) cold-pressed safflower or sunflower oil

Fruit filling (optional)
1 banana, sliced, or
1/2 cup (125 mL) berries (raspberries, strawberries, blueberries)
1 apple, chopped

Instructions
In a bowl, combine all pancake ingredients. Stir in optional fruit filling as desired. Spoon a dollop into heated (medium-heat) frying pan greased lightly with coconut oil or butter. When ready to flip, bubbles will begin to form on top. This basic mixture can also be used as waffle mix. Serves 2-3.

Yogurt Shake

Ingredients
1 cup (250 mL) plain probiotic yogurt
2 Tbsp (30 mL) flax meal
1 Tbsp (15 mL) EFA-oil blend (echium, borage, Udo's Choice oil,
    Omega Essential Balance oil, etc.)
1/2 cup (125 mL) fresh fruit of choice
1 cup (250 mL) organic fresh apple juice, diluted pomegranate juice, or juice of choice
3 ice cubes
Optional: 1-2 scoops protein powder (whey, pea, hemp, fermented soy)

Instructions
In a blender, combine all ingredients and blend until smooth. Drink immediately. Makes 1-2 servings.

For added heart support and blood sugar balancing, add in a serving of quality protein powder.

Appetizers, Dips, and Snacks

Black Bean Salsa

Ingredients

2 ripe tomatoes, chopped

1/4-1/2 cup (60-125 mL) chopped cilantro

1/3 cup (80 mL) finely chopped onion

1/3-3 serrano chili peppers

Salt to taste

1 can (15 oz/425 g) organic black beans, drained and rinsed

Juice of two limes

1/4 cup (60 mL) garlic-chili flaxseed oil (e.g., by Omega Nutrition)

Instructions

Place tomatoes in a medium bowl. Add the cilantro and onion to the tomatoes. Cut open the chilis, remove all the seeds, and dice very fine. Add chilis, salt, and beans to the tomato mixture. Pour lime juice and garlic-chili flaxseed oil over all ingredients. Mix, cover and refrigerate for one hour. Makes 3-4 cups (750 mL-1L).

Cilantro is an excellent detoxifying herb. It is specifically known to help the body excrete heavy metals, which is why holistic dentists advise patients who are having their mercury amalgams removed to eat lots of cilantro.

Much Maligned Avocado

Some physicians continue to warn heart patients and those on weight-reduction diets to avoid avocado. However, the avocado's bad rap is unjustified.

Superhero of the immune system, the avocado is rich in powerful detoxifier glutathione. Glutathione-rich avocados actually help cleanse the body of dangerous oxidized fats. Avocado has been wrongly dismissed as being unhealthy due to its fat content, but it contains monounsaturated fats, the ones we recommend to help the body deal with oxidation and free radicals.

Breezy California Rolls

Ingredients
3 cups (250 mL) brown rice, cooked
2 Tbsp (20 mL) rice wine vinegar
Nori (seaweed) sheets, one per roll
Handful of white sesame seeds
4 cups (1L) of vegetables of your choice, unless otherwise noted,
sliced into long, thin strips:

Avocado	Cucumber
Carrot	Zucchini, yellow or green
Lettuce, green or red, shredded	Peppers, red, yellow, or orange
Snow peas, whole or sliced lengthwise in two	

Optional: 1 cup (250 mL) cooked prawns, shrimp, soy tempeh, salmon, or any other mildly flavored fish

Instructions
You will need sushi rolling mats, which are reasonably priced at Asian supermarkets. You will need one mat per person rolling sushi.

To cooled brown rice, add the rice wine vinegar. As the rice cools, slice your vegetables (and protein) into matchstick shapes and set aside. Spread a nori sheet. On it, deposit a thin layer of rice, leaving a strip of nori bare at the top edge. Starting at the bottom, formulate a row of the vegetables (and seafood) of your choice. Toss on a few sesame seeds. Roll from the bottom and seal at the top by wetting the edge of seaweed with water. Slice into bite-size pieces and serve with minced ginger, wasabe, and organic soy sauce. Makes 12-16 rolls, depending on their thickness.

All ages love the make-do aspect of this recipe. Even grandchildren like to get into the act (under supervision, of course). Lay all the ingredients out on the table and let everybody create their own colorful versions.

Falafels in a Pita

One cup (250 mL) dry beans equals 2-2 1/2 cups (500-625 mL) cooked. You can soak and cook your own beans and put them in individual bags for future use. This is not only economical but makes for quick meals. Freezing soaked and cooked beans also makes them easier to digest and causes less gas and bloating.

Ingredients
4 cups (1 L) cooked garbanzo beans (also known as chick peas; they should be very soft)
6 cloves garlic, minced
1/2 cup (125 mL) finely chopped fresh parsley
1/2 cup (125 mL) finely minced onion
1 tsp (5 mL) cumin powder
Dash cayenne powder
2 eggs, beaten
4 Tbsp (60 mL) flax meal
2 Tbsp (30 mL) tahini (see recipe page 156)
2 Tbsp (30 mL) flour
5-10 whole wheat pita breads. This recipe
     makes 20-24 falafels, based on 2-4 per pita.
Pita Toppings: Tahini sauce (page 156), tsatziki (page 156), grated cheese, lettuce, tomato, onions, cucumber, and sprouts

Instructions
Using a food processor, mix garbanzo beans into a soft paste. Combine all ingredients except flour until well mixed. Refrigerate for at least one hour.

Lightly roll into balls, then roll in the flour and bake on a cookie sheet at 400°F (200°C) for 20-25 minutes or until crispy on the outside.

Place 2 to 4 falafels in a pita bread with tahini sauce (page 156) and/or tzatziki (page 156), grated cheese, lettuce, tomato, onions, cucumber, and sprouts. Makes 20-24 falafels.

Guacamole

Ingredients
3 ripe avocados, mashed
Juice of one small lemon
3 garlic cloves, pressed
1/2 cup (125 mL) chopped tomatoes
2 Tbsp (30 mL) finely minced green onion
2 Tbsp (30 mL) sour cream
3 Tbsp (45 mL) extra virgin olive oil

Instructions
Mix avocados with lemon juice and garlic. Mix thoroughly. I like using a fork to retain the dip's chunky texture. Add chopped tomatoes and green onion. Stir in sour cream and olive oil.

Serve as a condiment to fajitas or bean tortillas, with nachos, or as a layer in the Seven-layer Mexican Party Dip (see recipe below).

For a quick version, use 1/2 cup (125 mL) salsa in place of tomato and minced onion. Makes 4 servings.

Seven-layer Mexican Party Dip

Ingredients
2 cups (500 mL) refried beans (page 152)
1 cup (250 mL) white cheddar cheese
2 cups (500 mL) guacamole (above)
2 Tbsp (30 mL) finely chopped parsley
2 Tbsp (30 mL) finely chopped cilantro
1 cup (250 mL) full-fat organic yogurt
4 or 5 green onions, finely minced
2 tomatoes, chopped
1 bag organic-corn baked tortilla chips or whole-wheat crackers

Instructions
Preheat oven to 350°F (180°C). In a 9 in x 12 in (23 cm x 30 cm) glass baking dish, evenly spread the refried beans and cover with half of the grated cheese. Next, spread the guacamole, then sprinkle on the parsley and cilantro. Next, spread a layer of organic yogurt and green onions and then the chopped tomatoes. For the last layer, add the remaining grated cheese and sprinkle with parsley. Bake until the cheese melts and the dip is hot throughout. Serve at once with tortilla chips or crackers. Makes 6-8 servings.

Eggplant Dip

Ingredients
2 large eggplants
2 Tbsp (30 mL) tahini
1-2 garlic cloves, peeled and crushed
Juice of one medium lemon
Sea salt to taste

Instructions
Preheat oven to 350°F (180°C). Bake eggplants for 45 minutes. Remove from heat, allow to cool slightly, then, under cold running water, peel and discard eggplant skins. Let eggplant flesh drain in a colander for 10-15 minutes.

In a food processor, mix eggplants (taking care not to liquefy them too much), then stir in tahini, garlic, and lemon juice. Taste and add salt if required. Garnish with a sprig of mint or parsley. Makes 4 servings.

Eggplant is a vegetable that people often wonder how to incorporate into the diet. This recipe is very easy, and fibrous eggplant combined with protective garlic and the healthy fats in tahini make it wonderful heart food.

Hummus

Ingredients
2 cups (500 mL) cooked garbanzo beans (chickpeas) or 1 can
    (16 oz/500 mL), drained (save liquid)
4 garlic cloves, minced
3 Tbsp (45 mL) tahini (optional)
3 Tbsp (45 mL) extra virgin olive or flaxseed oil
1/3 cup (80 mL) freshly squeezed lemon juice
1/2 cup (250 mL) reserved liquid from chickpeas
1 tsp (5 mL) ground cumin
Salt to taste

Instructions
Put all ingredients in food processor and blend until smooth. If the hummus is too thick, add 2 Tbsp (30 mL) more oil and more lemon juice. Serve as a dip for vegetables or spread for whole-wheat crackers or whole-wheat pita bread. Makes 2 cups (500 mL).

Red Pepper Option: Brush 1 red pepper (halved) with olive oil and broil until soft and just starting to char. Allow to cool, then peel off the skin and add to blender with other ingredients.

Family Reunion Spinach Dip

Ingredients
1 package of prefrozen cooked spinach, defrosted
2/3 cup (170 mL) plain yogurt
1/4 cup (60 mL) mayonnaise (page 164)
1 8 oz can (225 mL) water chestnuts, chopped fine
1 Tbsp (15 mL) fresh chives, minced
2 cloves garlic, minced
Sea salt and pepper to taste
2 large, crusty whole grain round loaves
Optional: 1/4 cup (60 mL) black olives, chopped

Instructions
In a bowl, combine all ingredients and mix well, then chill. Just before serving, cut a bowl-shaped depression into the bread loaf, and fill with the dip. Around it on a serving tray, pile chunks of the inner bread and extra loaf as needed. Makes about 1 1/2 cups (375 mL) of dip.

Most families probably have a variation on this appetizer to whip up at birthdays and holidays. This version "cheats" on the side of health with fresh herbs and yogurt, and homemade mayonnaise.

Dressings

Lemon-garlic Dressing

Ingredients

2 garlic cloves, crushed

Juice of 1 lemon

Fresh herbs, crushed to taste (basil, coriander, mint)

4 Tbsp (60 mL) extra virgin olive oil

Sea salt to taste

Instructions

Chop garlic. Add lemon juice, herbs (if desired), and olive oil. Salt to taste. Add to salad just before serving. Makes 4 servings.

Flax-vinegar Favorite

Ingredients

2 garlic cloves, crushed

1 tsp (5 mL) mustard

3 Tbsp (45 mL) fresh lemon juice or organic apple cider vinegar

1/2 cup (125 mL) flaxseed oil

3 Tbsp (45 mL) water

1/2 tsp (2 mL) honey or maple syrup (optional)

Instructions

Put ingredients in blender and pureé together. Add to salad just before serving. Store remainder in air-sealed container in refrigerator for up to 1 week. Makes 3/4 cup (175 mL).

Multi-purpose Hearty Dressing

Ingredients

2 Tbsp (30 mL) olive oil

2 Tbsp (30 mL) Omega Nutrition garlic-chili flaxseed oil (or unflavored flaxseed oil)

1/2 cup (125 mL) apple cider vinegar

1 Tbsp (15 mL) organic apple cider or rice wine vinegar

2 Tbsp (30 mL) Dijon mustard (optional)

2 tsp (10 mL) brown sugar

Sea salt and freshly ground pepper to taste

Instructions

Combine all ingredients in a jar. Briskly stir and serve over any vegetable/grain salad. Serves 3-4.

Marvellously Easy Miso Dressing

Ingredients
2 Tbsp (30 mL) miso paste
2 tsp (10 mL) dried onions
2 Tbsp (30 mL) organic apple cider vinegar
1 Tbsp (15 mL) manuka honey
1/4 cup (60 mL) olive oil
1/2 cup (125 mL) water

Optional: A handful of sesame seeds, or freshly grated ginger to taste.

Instructions
Combine all ingredients and serve over salad of your choice. Refrigerate leftover dressing for up to 2 weeks. Makes about 1 cup (250 mL).

Sweet Poppy Seed Salad Dressing

Ingredients
4 Tbsp (60 mL) manuka honey
1/3 cup (80 mL) organic apple cider vinegar
1 Tbsp (15 mL) lemon juice
1 Tbsp (15 mL) poppy seeds
Handful of dried currants (optional)

Instructions
Mix all ingredients together, and serve over chilled green salad. Store unused dressing in the fridge up to 1 week. Makes about 2/3 cup (160 mL).

You will find manuka honey at health food stores; this New Zealand import has been studied for its impressive antibacterial properties. It is, at therapeutic potency, even used to treat wounds and infections.

♥ Easty-to-use Grated Ginger

Here is a quick tip for using ginger. Buy ginger, wash it, dry it, then store it in the freezer in a resealable plastic bag. Grate it straight from the freezer as needed. It will not go bad.

Salads

Tofu Tempeh Salad with Curry

Ingredients
2 packages of tempeh (fermented soy curd), steamed, crumbled
2-3 Tbsp (30-45 mL) parsley, chopped
2-3 Tbsp (30-45 mL) cilantro, finely chopped
1/4 cup (60 mL) celery, chopped
1/4 cup (60 mL) nuts of your choice
1/4 cup (60 mL) dried fruits (optional)
1 tsp (5 mL) turmeric
1 tsp (5 mL) masala (spice of coriander, cinnamon, cardamom, cumin)
1 tsp (5 mL) organic, wheat-free tamari
1/4 cup (60 mL) plain yogurt

Instructions
Toss all ingredients together in a large bowl. Spoon onto a bed of lettuce and serve. Makes 3-4 servings.

Spinach, Strawberry, and Feta Salad

Ingredients
1 bunch (500 mL) fresh spinach
1/2 cup (125 mL) strawberries, sliced
1/2 cup (125 mL) almonds, slivered
1/2 cup (125 mL) carrot, finely shredded
1/4 cup (60 mL) feta cheese

Dressing
2 Tbsp (15 mL) honey
1/4 cup (60 mL) organic apple cider vinegar
1/2 cup (125 mL) extra virgin olive oil

Instructions
In a medium bowl, toss spinach, strawberries, almonds, and carrots. Mix together dressing ingredients. Pour dressing over salad, toss, and serve immediately. Makes 4 servings.

Marinated Broccoli and Cherry Tomato Salad

This recipe should be made several hours before serving to allow the dressing to flavor the vegetables and soften the broccoli.

Ingredients
2 cups (500 mL) bean sprouts
1 medium red pepper, sliced
3 cups (750 mL) chopped broccoli, cut into bite-size pieces
1 small red onion, thinly sliced
1 cup (250 mL) halved cherry tomatoes
1/2-3/4 cup (125-180 mL) pistachio nut oil or vegetarian
    EFA-rich oil, or extra-virgin olive oil
2 Tbsp (30 mL) organic apple cider vinegar (or to taste)
6 Tbsp (90 mL) organic, wheat-free tamari
2 garlic cloves, pressed
1/4 cup (60 mL) black sesame seeds

Instructions
Combine sprouts, red pepper, broccoli, onion, and cherry tomatoes in a large serving bowl. Combine the oil, vinegar, tamari, and garlic in a container and shake well. Pour dressing over salad and toss well. Garnish with black sesame seeds. Cover and refrigerate until serving, tossing occasionally. Makes 6 servings.

"Catherine the Great" Salad

Ingredients
2 cups (500 mL) brown rice or other whole grain, cooked
1 cup (250 mL) mixed sprouts
1/2 cup (125 mL) fresh herbs, chopped (parsley, cilantro, dill)
1 medium tomato, chopped
1 cucumber, chopped
2-3 garlic cloves, minced
Juice of one lemon
1/4 cup (60 mL) extra virgin olive oil
Sea salt and black pepper to taste

Instructions
Combine rice and salad vegetables in a medium bowl. Mix garlic, lemon juice, olive oil, sea salt, and black pepper in a dish. Drizzle over salad, toss, and enjoy. Makes 4-6 servings.

Avocado and Sweet Nut Salad

Ingredients
1/4 cup (60 mL) green cabbage, sliced
1/4 cup (60 mL) celery, chopped finely
1/2 cup (125 mL) spinach, torn into bite-size pieces
1 ripe pear, sliced thinly
1 ripe avocado, sliced
3 fresh figs, peeled and sliced (optional)
1/4 cup (60 mL) chopped walnuts, almonds, or cashews

Dressing
2 Tbsp (30 mL) extra virgin olive oil
1 Tbsp (15 mL) manuka honey
1 tsp (5 mL) lemon juice

Instructions
On a serving plate, layer the cabbage, celery, and spinach, then the pears, avocado, and figs (if desired). Add the chopped nuts last and drizzle in dressing just before serving. Makes 2-3 servings.

Shrimp and Sugar Snap Pea Salad

Ingredients
Shrimp mixture
36 large shrimp, deveined, shelled
     and lightly steamed until cooked
1 cup (250 mL) sugar snap peas
     or snow peas with ends removed
1 cucumber, thinly sliced
1/4 cup (60 mL) finely chopped parsley
2 thinly sliced celery stalks

Dressing
5 Tbsp (75 mL) EFA-rich oil blend or hazelnut oil
1/4 cup (60 mL) apple cider vinegar
1 Tbsp (15 mL) toasted sesame oil
4 Tbsp (60 mL) organic, wheat-free tamari
1 Tbsp (15 mL) Dijon mustard
1 Tbsp (15 mL) honey
Course ground black pepper
Sea salt to taste

Salad bed
3 1/2-4 cups (875 mL-1L) cooked whole-wheat couscous, or fresh wild mixed greens

Instructions
In a large bowl, combine shrimp, peas, cucumber, parsley, and celery. Mix dressing ingredients and pour over shrimp mixture. Refrigerate for two hours. Place couscous or greens on a serving dish and arrange shrimp mixture on top. Makes 6-8 servings.

Mint-fresh Cucumber Salad

Ingredients
4 medium cucumbers, sliced and peeled
1/4 cup (60 mL) organic apple cider vinegar
Juice of half a lemon
Half a bunch of parsley, finely chopped
Half a bunch of mint, finely chopped
3/4 cup (180 mL) plain yogurt

Instructions
Mix everything together and chill before serving. Makes 4-6 servings.

Mediterranean Tabouleh Salad

Ingredients
2 cups (500 mL) bulgur wheat, cooked
4 medium tomatoes, chopped
2-3 green onions, chopped fine
1/2 bunch parsley with stalks, chopped
1/4 cup (60 mL) extra virgin olive oil
Juice of 1 large or 2 small lemons

Instructions
In a bowl, add cooled wheat and all ingredients. Allow to chill in fridge (ideally overnight), and serve cold. Makes 4 servings.

Artichoke Greek Salad

Ingredients
3 ripe tomatoes, medium size, chopped
1 large cucumber, chopped
2 (14 oz) jars of artichoke hearts, drained, chopped
Black olives, as many or as few as you want
1/4 cup (60 mL) extra virgin olive oil
3 Tbsp (45 mL) balsamic vinegar
1 tsp (5 mL) dried oregano
1/2 cup (125 mL) feta cheese (optional)

Instructions
Toss tomatoes, cucumber, artichokes, and olives into a medium bowl. In a small jar, mix olive oil, vinegar, dried oregano, and (optional) some artichoke jar juice. Mix dressing, then pour over vegetables and toss. If desired, crumble feta cheese over the top. Best served chilled. Makes 4 servings.

Greek salad is one of those dishes that is guaranteed to please. I like adding the artichoke hearts for a bit more originality and color.

Soupy Stuff

Traditional Japanese Miso *Shi-ru* with Vegetables

This *shi-ru* (soup) is surprisingly easy, quick, and irresistibly tasty. You can buy dehydrated miso soup vegetables and mixes at most Asian markets. Root vegetables are very popular in Japan, especially in the fall. You can also buy pre-prepared root veggie combinations, usually stored in the refrigerated section.

Ingredients
Your choice of 1 1/2 cups (375 mL) sliced vegetables

Carrot, pre-steamed	Celery, pre-steamed
Parsnip, pre-steamed	Daikon radish, sliced fine
Lotus root	Burdock root, cooked
Dried mushrooms	Dried onions
Dried seaweed	

Chunks of precooked fish, shrimp, prawns, clams, or mussels (optional)
1/4 cup (60 mL) miso paste (keep stored in your fridge)

Instructions
Bring 6 cups (1.5L) of water to a boil in a medium pot, then reduce heat. Add your vegetables, dried ingredients, and (optional) seafood and simmer on low.

In a small bowl, mix your miso with enough water to make it slightly soupy (this will prevent later clumping). Add miso mixture to the still warm (but not boiling) water. (Boiling miso destroys beneficial enzymes and flavor.) Serve immediately. Makes 4-6 servings.

Serve with fresh greens with your choice of dressings and/or sliced cucumber topped with miso paste.

Black Bean Soup

Ingredients
2 cups (500 mL) chopped onion
6 garlic cloves, minced
2 tsp (10 mL) ground cumin
2 tsp (10 mL) coriander
4 Tbsp (60 mL) olive oil
2 cans (14 oz/400 g) black beans (or 2 cups/500 mL of dry beans soaked and cooked
    in 4 cups/1L of water)
2 cups (500 mL) vegetable stock or puréed tomatoes
1/2 cup (125 mL) chopped red pepper
1/2 cup (125 mL) finely chopped parsley
1/2 cup (125 mL) chopped cilantro
1/8 tsp (0.5 mL) cayenne pepper
Juice of medium freshly squeezed lemon
1/2 cup (125 mL) EFA-rich oil blend
Chopped green onions, cilantro, yogurt for garnish

Instructions
In a large, heavy-bottomed pot, sauté onions, garlic, cumin, and coriander in olive oil until onions are soft. Add beans, vegetable stock or puréed tomatoes, red pepper, parsley, and cilantro. Simmer over medium heat for 30 minutes. Purée soup in blender or use a hand-held blender in the soup pot. If the soup is too thick, add a little more stock, juice, and EFA-rich oil blend.

Serve garnished with chopped green onions, cilantro, and a dollop of yogurt. This soup can be frozen without the garnishes. Makes 6 servings.

Lentil Carrot Soup

Ingredients
6 cups (1.5L) vegetable stock
1 bay leaf
2 1/2 cups (625 mL) raw lentils
2 cups (500 mL) chopped carrots
1 1/2 cups (375 mL) chopped onions
1 cup (250 mL) chopped celery
6 garlic cloves, crushed
1 cup (250 mL) diced potato or yam
1 tsp (5 mL) ground cumin
1/2 tsp (2 mL) oregano
Black pepper to taste
2 cups (500 mL) diced fresh tomatoes
1/4 cup (60 mL) red wine
1/4 cup (60 mL) EFA-oil rich blend (e.g., borage, echium, Omega's Essential Balance)
1/2 cup (125 mL) chopped parsley
1/2 cup (125 mL) minced green onions and parsley for garnish

Instructions
Simmer vegetable stock, bay leaf, and lentils for 4 to 5 hours. In a separate pan, sauté carrots, onions, celery, garlic, potato, herbs, and spices. Add to lentil mixture and simmer for 15 minutes. Add tomatoes and red wine and simmer until vegetables are cooked to desired tenderness. Remove bay leaf before serving.

Remove from heat and stir in EFA-rich oil blend. Garnish with chopped parsley and green onions. Serve with thickly sliced whole wheat bread. Makes 6 servings.

The longer this soup simmers, the better. We find the process of making it, smelling it, stirring it occasionally, almost therapeutic. There is something relaxing about a day spent nurturing a simmering pot.

Traditional Tomato Soup

Ingredients
2 Tbsp (30 mL) butter
1 medium onion, chopped
1/2 cup leek stalk (125 mL), chopped
2 garlic cloves, chopped
2 jars (2 - 350 mL) of tomatoes
1 tsp (5 mL) brown sugar
Pinch of baking soda
Sea salt and black pepper to taste

Instructions
Heat butter in a medium-size saucepan. Add onion, leek, fresh garlic and sauté until the onion is soft and translucent. Add tomatoes and liquid from both jars. Blend with a hand blender. Add sugar, baking soda, and seasoning. Simmer for 15-20 minutes on low heat. Garnish with a dollop of sour cream and sprigs of parsley. Makes 6 servings.

♥ Choose Tomatoes in Glass

Whenever possible, use fresh vine-ripened tomatoes. As a second choice, use tomatoes preserved in glass containers. The acidity of tomatoes can eat away at the inner, bisphenol-A plastic coating of the typical can. As you may know, bisphenol-A is a toxic, hormone-disrupting chemical. Avoid purchasing canned tomato products.

Classic Minestrone Soup

Ingredients
6 garlic cloves, crushed
2 cups (500 mL) chopped onion
1 cup (250 mL) sliced celery
4 Tbsp (60 mL) extra virgin olive oil
2 cups (500 mL) sliced carrots
1 cup (250 mL) chopped red pepper
Sea salt or mineralized salt to taste
1/4 cup (60 mL) finely chopped cilantro
2 bay leaves
2 tsp (10 mL) fresh oregano
2 tsp (10 mL) fresh basil
4 cups (1L) stock soup (use nonhydrolized vegetable bouillon cubes)
1 can (14 oz/400 g) garbanzo or pinto beans, drained and rinsed
2 cups (500 mL) tomato purée
1 1/2 cups (375 mL) chopped fresh tomatoes
1/4 cup (60 mL) dry red wine
1/2 cup (125 mL) dry whole wheat pasta, cooked firm and set aside
1/2 cup (125 mL) EFA-rich oil blend
Freshly grated parmesan cheese, for garnish
Freshly ground coarse black pepper, for garnish
1 cup (250 mL) finely chopped parsley, for garnish

Instructions
Fizzle garlic, onions, and celery in olive oil in a large, heavy-bottomed soup pot. Add carrots, red peppers, salt, and fresh herbs. Cover and simmer for 5 minutes. Add stock, beans, tomato purée, tomatoes, and red wine. Cover and simmer on low heat for 20 minutes. Remove bay leaves.

Add pasta. Cook until tender. Remove from heat, stir in EFA-rich oil blend, and top with freshly grated Parmesan cheese, black pepper, and parsley. Makes 8 servings.

Split Pea *Sans* Ham Soup

Ingredients
1 1/2 cups (375 mL) split peas, dried
1/2 cup (125 mL) barley
6 1/2 cups (1.75L) water
1 stalk of celery, chopped finely
1 large carrot, chopped finely
1 leek, chopped finely
1 potato, diced
1 bay leaf
1/2 tsp each or to taste of dried thyme, basil, cumin, marjoram, and ground black pepper
1 tsp (5 mL) sea salt

Instructions
Put all ingredients into a large pot. Bring to a boil, then simmer on low heat for 3 or more hours. Makes 6 servings.

Ratatouille

Ingredients
1 large onion, coarsely chopped
6 garlic cloves, minced
2 Tbsp (30 mL) water
4 Tbsp (60 mL) olive oil
1 small eggplant, cubed
1 cup (250 mL) tomato sauce
1 bay leaf
1 tsp (5 mL) fresh basil
1 tsp (5 ml) oregano
1/8 tsp (0.5 mL) finely chopped rosemary
1 large zucchini, cubed
1 medium red pepper, cubed (seeds removed)
1 medium green pepper, cubed (seeds removed)
3 large tomatoes, coarsely chopped
3 Tbsp (45 mL) tomato paste
1/2 cup (125 mL) EFA-rich oil blend
1/2 cup (125 mL) chopped parsley

Instructions
In a large, deep pot, frizzle onion and garlic in water and olive oil (be careful of spitting) until onion turns translucent. Add eggplant, tomato sauce, bay leaf, basil, oregano, and rosemary. Mix ingredients, cover, and simmer on low heat for 20 minutes. Stir in zucchini and red and green peppers and simmer for another 5 minutes. Stir in tomatoes and tomato paste.

Mix thoroughly. Simmer until vegetables are cooked to desired tenderness. Turn off the heat and stir in EFA-rich oil blend and chopped parsley.

Add some good hearty whole-grain or whole-wheat bread and a side-dish of brown basmati rice. Makes 6 servings.

Dr. Ron's Vegetarian Chili

Ingredients
2 large onions, finely chopped
8 garlic cloves, minced
1 small jalapeno pepper, finely chopped (optional)
3 tsp (15 mL) chili powder (more if you like it hot)
2 tsp (10 mL) cumin powder
2 tsp (10 mL) coriander powder
Sea salt and pepper to taste
1/4 tsp (1 mL) cayenne pepper
1 cup (250 mL) finely chopped celery
1/4 cup (60 mL) extra virgin olive oil
2-4 Tbsp (30-60 mL) water
2 cups (500 mL) grated carrots
2 cups (500 mL) grated zucchini
1 large red pepper, chopped
1 large green pepper, chopped
2 cups (500 mL) fresh tomatoes, chopped
1 jar (16 oz/500 g) stewed tomatoes
1 jar (16 oz/500 g) tomato sauce
1 can (14 oz/400 g) kidney beans, drained and rinsed
1 can (14 oz/400 g) pinto beans, drained and rinsed
1/2 cup (125 mL) EFA-rich oil blend

Instructions
In a very deep, heavy-bottomed-pan, sauté (over low to medium heat) the onions, garlic, jalapeno pepper, spices, and celery in the olive oil and water until soft. Add carrots, zucchini, and chopped red and green peppers. Frizzle for 5-10 minutes, stirring occasionally. Add more water if needed to keep veggies from sticking. Add the fresh and stewed tomatoes, and sauce. Add beans.

Turn down heat to minimum and let simmer for several hours. Remove from heat and add EFA-rich oil blend just before serving. It is great when served with warm, hearty buns and a dollop of whole-fat organic yogurt or grated sharp cheese. Makes 6 servings.

Vegetables

If broccoli and cauliflower mark the extent of your vegetable creativity, we encourage you to visit farmers markets and experiment. Often, the vendor will be familiar with cooking unfamiliar vegetables — especially greens — so don't be afraid to ask. The more diversity of foods you eat, the healthier it is, supplying your body with important anti-aging, disease-fighting nutrients and cofactors.

Fabulous Gingered Asparagus or Green Beans

Ingredients
3/4 cup (180 mL) apple cider vinegar
1 1/2 Tbsp (25 mL) freshly grated gingerroot
2 Tbsp (30 mL) organic maple syrup
1 lb (500 g) fresh asparagus or green beans
2 garlic cloves, minced
3-4 Tbsp (45-60 mL) sesame oil
1/2 tsp (2 mL) sea salt
1 tsp (5 mL) organic tamari

Instructions
Combine vinegar, grated gingerroot, and maple syrup and bring to a boil. Cook uncovered over medium heat for 10-15 minutes to make a deep ginger-tasting sauce and set aside.

Cut off 1/2 in (1.5 cm) from base of asparagus, or clip off ends of green beans. Steam until tender, about 5-8 minutes. Remove from heat and rinse with cold water to stop the cooking.

Combine garlic, oil, sea salt, and tamari with vinegar mixture. Arrange asparagus or green beans on a plate. Cover with marinade and refrigerate for 1 or 2 hours before serving. Makes 4 servings.

Baked Spaghetti Squash

Ingredients
1 spaghetti squash, deseeded and quartered
Dash of cinnamon
Sea salt and pepper to taste
Dollop of butter, coconut oil

Instructions
On a baking sheet, set 4 pieces of squash face up. Sprinkle with cinnamon. Add a small dollop of butter or coconut oil onto each piece (optional). Bake in preheated oven at 400°F (200°C) and bake for approx 15-20 minutes. Once squash has softened (you should be able to peel away squash strands with a fork), remove from oven and serve with skin on.

Just before serving, another option is to drizzle lightly with an EFA-rich oil blend, or garlic/chili flax oil. Makes 4-6 servings.

Seasoned Broccoli Sauté

Ingredients
1 pound broccoli or broccoli rabe, trimmed
1 clove garlic, minced
1 Tbsp (15 mL) extra virgin olive oil
1 Tbsp (15 mL) tamari sauce (optional)
1-2 Tbsp (15-30 mL) Parmesan cheese, grated (optional)

Instructions
Bring a pot of salted water to a boil and cook broccoli until just tender, then set aside. In a pan, sauté garlic in olive oil. Add broccoli and sauté for another 5-8 minutes, then scoop onto a serving plate and sprinkle with tamari or Parmesan cheese. Makes 4 servings.

Made-in-Minutes Sautéed Greens

Ingredients
Your choice or combination of green leafy vegetables — kale, chard,
    bok choi, beet greens, dandelion, and spinach ripped or cut into
    bite-size pieces
Dollop of butter or coconut oil (optional)
1 medium onion, sliced
2-3 cloves of garlic, thinly sliced
Grated ginger (optional: for ginger tip, see page 130)
Sea salt and pepper to taste

Instructions
In a sauté pan, melt 1 Tbsp (15 mL) of butter or coconut oil. Sauté onion and garlic
(and ginger, if desired) on medium heat until almost cooked. Add enough water to
cover the bottom of the skillet and the greens of your choice. Cover with a lid, stirring
occasionally until cooked. Serve warm, seasoned to taste. Makes 4 servings.

Option: Use water and 2 Tbsp (30 mL) of tamari sauce when you sauté your vegetable
of choice.

Thyme-to-Make Zucchini

Ingredients
2 small green zucchini, chopped
2 small yellow zucchini, chopped
1 Tbsp (15 mL) extra virgin olive oil (optional)
Sprigs of thyme, oregano, or savory
2 tsp (10 mL) lemon

Instructions
In a large skillet, sauté zucchini in olive oil (or use water) over low-medium heat. Add
herb sprigs and lemon juice. Cook for 2-3 more minutes until tender. Makes 4 servings.

Oil-less Vegetable Stir-Frizzle

Any combination of your favorite vegetables will work with this recipe.

Ingredients
1 cup (250 mL) vegetable stock
3-4 Tbsp (45-60 mL) organic tamari
3 garlic cloves, pressed
1 Tbsp (15 mL) peeled and finely sliced fresh ginger
1 tsp (5 mL) sesame oil (for flavor only)
1 large onion, coarsely chopped
1 medium head of broccoli, cut into bite-size pieces
1 carrot, sliced diagonally
1 red pepper, coarsely chopped
1/2 cup (125 mL) pistachio oil, or EFA-rich blend (Udo's Choice, echium,
     borage, Omega's Essential Balance), or hazelnut oil

Instructions
In a wok or very large pot, combine stock, tamari, garlic, ginger, and sesame oil. Heat liquid and then add all the vegetables except the red pepper. Cook until veggies are tender-firm, then add the red pepper. Cover and cook to the desired tenderness. Remove from heat and stir in the oil you chose. Serve with brown rice and Excellent Ginger Sauce (page 155). Makes 2-4 servings.

♥ Skip the Non-stick Pan

Non-stick cookware may seem convenient and easy to clean, but is it safe? Not if it is coated with the toxic Teflon chemical perfluorooctanoic acid (PFOA). PFOA accumulates in the body and harms development, immune function, and hormone health. PFOA and other Teflon-family chemicals have also been linked to several types of cancer, including that of the liver, pancreas, and testes.

Cookware made from stainless steel, titanium, cast iron, enamelled cast-iron (lead- and cadmium-free), and glass are safer kitchen options. Le Creuset pans with the matte black enamel interior are fabulous. The company makes its matte black and white interior enamel from the same material, but the black interior is fired at a higher temperature and withstands higher cooking temperatures. You will love the Le Creuset pan — clean up is a breeze.

For more information on Teflon chemicals, visit the Environmental Working Group at www.ewg.org.

Main Dishes

As Good As It Gets Pizza (Spelt Crust)

Toppings
Your choice of chopped peppers, mushrooms, onions, olives, zucchini, broccoli, tomatoes (sun-dried or sliced), green onions, artichokes, baked chicken breast, precooked shrimp, precooked scallops, pine nuts, pineapple, or ... anything goes! Get creative.

Pizza crust
1 cup (250 mL) warm water
1 Tbsp (15 mL) quick rise yeast
2 1/2 cups (625 mL) spelt flour
1 tsp (5 mL) sea salt
1/4 cup (60 mL) extra virgin olive oil

Instructions
Mix water and yeast in a cup. To a large bowl containing the spelt flour and salt, add the water-yeast mixture. Knead in the olive oil. Allow dough to rise for about an hour (it will double in size) by covering with a clean towel and placing somewhere warm. Pound down the risen dough, then place somewhere warm again for about 30 minutes. Then spread over pizza sheet, pile high with vegetables and protein of your choice, and cook in an oven preheated to 400°F (200°C) for 20-30 minutes or until warm and golden brown. Crust recipe makes 2 medium pizzas.

Herb-infused Halibut or Swordfish

Ingredients
1 pound (500 g) halibut or swordfish, in four pieces
1/2 cup (125 mL) fresh herbs of your choice, chopped
Good choices include: Thyme, rosemary, dill, savory, marjoram, basil, or oregano
Sea salt and pepper
3 Tbsp (15 mL) extra virgin olive oil

Instructions
Dip fish pieces into mixed herbs, salt, and pepper. Wrap in aluminum foil and refrigerate for an hour to infuse. Remove from the fridge, drizzle with oil and grill over low-medium heat. Squeeze fresh lemon or lime over fish immediately before serving. Makes 4 servings.

Cauliflower Curry

Ingredients
Curry sauce
1 tsp (5 mL) coriander
1 tsp (5 mL) cumin powder
1/4 tsp (1 mL) ground cloves
4 garlic cloves, peeled
1 tsp (5 mL) peeled and grated fresh gingerroot
1/2 tsp (2 mL) turmeric
1/8 – 1/4 tsp (0.5-1 mL) cayenne pepper
1/2 cup (125 mL) water

Cauliflower mixture
2 cups (500 mL) onion, coarsely chopped
1 large cauliflower, cut into bite-size pieces (sliced yams and cubed
     potatoes can be added for variation)
Juice of 1 lemon
3 Tbsp (45 mL) pistachio nut oil

Instructions
Mix sauce ingredients in blender or food processor, or with a whisk, until well blended.
Set aside.

Sauté onions on low heat in olive oil and 2 Tbsp (30 mL) of water until soft. Add
cauliflower (or other vegetables). Add sauce mixture and cook covered, on low heat, until
cauliflower (or other vegetables) are tender but not soft. Once cooked, remove from heat.
Stir in lemon juice and pistachio nut oil.

Serve with brown rice, veggies, and plain yogurt. Sprinkle with toasted sesame
seeds. Makes 4 servings.

Refried Beans (Frijoles Refritos)

Ingredients
2 cans (16 oz/454 g) black beans or pinto beans
1 large onion, finely chopped
3 Tbsp (45 mL) extra virgin olive oil
4 garlic cloves, minced
1 tsp (5 mL) coriander
1 tsp (5 mL) ground cumin
1/2 cup (125 mL) salsa
1/4 cup (60 mL) chopped fresh cilantro
2 Tbsp (3 mL) EFA-rich oil blend
1 cup grated cheese (optional)

Instructions
Drain the cans of beans, reserving the liquid from one can. Set aside. (If you get gas from eating beans, then discard all the liquid and rinse the beans.)

In a deep skillet, frizzle onion with olive oil, garlic, coriander, and cumin until onion is soft. Slowly add beans, 1/2 cup (125 mL) at a time. Mash the beans with a potato masher. Add salsa and chopped cilantro. Heat thoroughly.

Remove from heat and stir in EFA-rich oil blend. Top with grated cheese and serve as a main course with a green salad. Makes 6 servings.

Fassoulia (Beans)

Ingredients
4 cups (1 L) large lima beans, cooked
1 cup (250 mL) leeks, chopped
2 Tbsp (30 mL) extra virgin olive oil
1 cup (250 mL) fresh or jarred tomatoes

Instructions
With cooked lima beans set to the side, sauté leeks in olive oil for a few minutes. Add tomatoes and lima beans until leeks are tender. Add sea salt and pepper to taste and serve immediately with a salad and a hearty bread. Makes 4 servings.

Option: Switch lima beans for sliced zucchini. Add basil and oregano to taste during cooking and serve as an accompanying dish.

Southwest Chicken and Black Bean Pasta

Ingredients
1/2 cup (125 mL) extra virgin olive oil
4 garlic cloves, minced
2 lbs (1 kg) chicken tenders* (tendon removed)
1 medium onion, chopped
1 red pepper, diced
1/2 cup (125 mL) chopped fresh cilantro
1/2 cup (125 mL) chopped fresh parsley
1/8 tsp (0.5 mL) cayenne pepper
1 can (16 oz/500 g) black beans, drained and rinsed
1 jar (6 oz/180 mL) tomato paste
1 jar (16 oz/500 g) stewed tomatoes or 8 large
    fresh tomatoes, chopped
6 Tbsp (90 mL) garlic-chili flaxseed oil
16 oz (500 g) cooked whole grain pasta
Freshly grated Parmesan cheese, for garnish
Freshly ground pepper, for garnish

Instructions
In a deep pan, slowly sauté olive oil, garlic, chicken, and onions on low heat until thoroughly cooked. Add red pepper, cilantro, parsley, cayenne, and black beans. Cook until heated. Then add the tomato paste and stewed tomatoes. Simmer for 5 minutes. Remove from heat and add garlic-chili flaxseed oil. Stir thoroughly, then serve with cooked, drained pasta. Serve hot and garnished with Parmesan cheese and freshly ground pepper. Makes 6 servings.

* Strip of muscle that runs along the inside of the breast closest to the bone.

Fish with Zesty Orange Glaze

Ingredients
1 Tbsp (15 mL) butter or coconut oil
4 fish steaks or fillets of your choice
Sea salt and pepper
3 Tbsp (45 mL) tamari sauce or soy sauce
Juice of one orange
1/2 tsp (2.5 mL) sesame or walnut oil
     or
Handful of sesame seeds or crumbled walnuts

Instructions
In a frying pan, melt 1 Tbsp (15 mL) butter or coconut oil. Cook fish dressed with salt and pepper over medium heat until lightly browned on both sides. Remove fish and set in warmer. Add tamari or soy sauce with orange juice to the frying pan and turn to high heat, stirring constantly. Once mixture has glazed, add sesame or walnut oil, or sesame seeds or walnuts. Drizzle over still warm fish and serve at once. Makes 4 servings.

Spicy Pepper Scallops

Ingredients
2 cups (500 g) colored peppers, thinly sliced
1 cup (250 g) red onion, thinly sliced
1 pound (500 g) scallops
1 Tbsp (15 mL) tamari sauce
1 tsp (5 mL) hot sesame oil
Black sesame seeds (optional)

Instructions
In a hot wok, stirfry vegetables in a few tablespoons (30-45 mL) of water over medium-high heat, making sure to stir constantly so the veggies don't burn. If needed, splash in a bit more water. After about 5 minutes, remove from heat and set aside. Vegetables should be just cooked.

Stirfry scallops in heated wok in leftover water/veggie juice for a few minutes, then re-toss with your vegetables. Add the tamari and hot sesame oil. Cook covered for another minute or two. Serve immediately onto plates and garnish with black sesame seeds. Makes 4 servings.

Condiments

Excellent Ginger Sauce

This sauce is delicious with rice, Chinese vegetables, chicken, or seafood.

Ingredients
1/2 cup (125 mL) onion, finely chopped
2 Tbsp (30 mL) gingerroot, peeled and grated or finely sliced
3 garlic cloves, minced
2 Tbsp (30 mL) extra virgin olive oil or hazelnut oil
1/2 cup (125 mL) organic, wheat-free tamari or soy sauce
1/2 cup (125 mL) water
2 tsp (10 mL) organic apple cider vinegar
1 Tbsp (15 mL) cornstarch
2 Tbsp (30 mL) EFA-rich oil blend (e.g. borage, echium, Udo's Choice)

Instructions
In a saucepan on low heat, frizzle onion, gingerroot, and garlic in olive oil. Combine tamari (or soy sauce), water, apple cider vinegar, and cornstarch. Whisk until well mixed. Add mixture to saucepan and stir until sauce thickens, about 3 to 5 minutes. Remove from heat and stir in EFA-rich oil blend. Refrigerate in an airtight container. Makes 2 cups (500 mL).

Cheese-free Sauce with a Kick

Ingredients
2 small potatoes, chopped
1 carrot, chopped
3 cups (750 ml) water
1 tsp (5 mL) sea salt
1 Tbsp (15 mL) Dijon mustard
Chopped or dried herbs such as parsley, garlic, or chives (optional)
Pepper to taste

Instructions
Cook potatoes and carrot in water until tender. Put vegetables, water, salt, and Dijon mustard into a blender and blend until smooth. Add herbs if desired. Serve warm, peppered to taste, over vegetables, pasta, or grains. Makes about 3 cups (750 mL).

Tahini Sauce

Ingredients
1 cup (250 mL) tahini
1/2 cup (125 mL) freshly squeezed lemon juice
1/2 - 1 cup (125-250 mL) water
4 garlic cloves
1 Tbsp (15 mL) organic tamari
4 Tbsp (60 mL) extra virgin olive oil

Instructions
Combine all ingredients in a blender and process until smooth. Refrigerate. Serve with vegetables, chicken, falafels, or other dippy foods. Makes 1 1/2 cups (375 mL).

Tzatziki (Cucumber Yogurt) Sauce

Ingredients
1 cup (250 mL) plain yogurt
1/2 cup (125 mL) grated cucumber
4 Tbsp (60 mL) extra virgin olive oil
2 Tbsp (30 mL) onion, finely minced
2 garlic cloves, minced

Instructions
Combine all ingredients. Chill for one hour. Serve with vegetables, chicken, falafels, or other dippy foods. Makes 1 1/2 cups (375 mL).

This is one of our summertime favorites, when the cucumber is local and the company for dinner always plentiful. The yogurt provides a cooling touch that meshes nicely with anything off the barbecue.

Quick and Easy Pesto

Make plenty when basil is in season and freeze it for all-year cooking.

Ingredients
3 cups (750 mL) packed, fresh basil leaves, washed, dried, and with thick stems removed
4-6 garlic cloves, peeled
1/2 cup (125 mL) pine nuts
1/2 cup (125 mL) freshly grated Parmesan cheese
1/2 cup (125 mL) EFA-rich oil blend, or hazelnut oil, or flaxseed oil

Instructions
Put basil leaves, garlic, pine nuts, Parmesan cheese, and half of the oil into the food processor and blend until ingredients are well mixed. While the processor is still running, pour in the remaining oil. Pesto will become a thick paste. Keep sealed in refrigerator and use within one day or basil will oxidize and turn black. Cook your favorite whole-grain pasta and serve together. Makes 2 cups (500 mL).

Variations on Basil Pesto
Sun-dried Tomato Pesto: Replace half the basil with a 2 oz (60 g) jar of sun-dried tomatoes (oil drained).

Roasted Red Pepper Pesto: Replace half the basil with two large roasted red peppers. To roast red peppers, place on baking sheet in a 250°F (120°C) oven for 25 minutes. Turn twice during cooking. Remove from oven and leave to cool on a wire rack. When cool, peel skin and remove seeds.

Roasted red peppers are excellent as a side dish with a splash of garlic-chili flaxseed oil.

Desserts and Baked Stuff

Herbed Biscuits

Ingredients
2 cups (500 mL) whole wheat flour
2 1/2 cups (625 mL) flour, unbleached
2 tsp (10 mL) sea salt
4 tsp (20 mL) baking powder
3 Tbsp (45 mL) chives, minced
3 Tbsp (45 mL) parsley, minced
3/4 cup (180 mL) extra virgin olive oil
2 cups (500 mL) milk or milk substitute

Instructions
Lightly grease two cookie sheets with butter or coconut oil. Mix together the flours, sea salt, and baking powder in a large bowl. In a smaller bowl, combine olive oil and milk or milk substitute. Add wet ingredients to dry ingredients and stir until well mixed. Using a tablespoon, scoop mixture onto cookie sheets and bake for 12-15 minutes at 350°F (180°C). Bottoms will be brown when done. Remove from heat and cool on a wire rack.

Makes about 2 dozen biscuits.

All-fruit Frozen Dessert (or Popsicles)

This recipe is perfect when berries are in season and you are buying extra to store in the freezer anyway. You can use any fruit combination you want — bananas, oranges, berries, mango, or pineapple.

Ingredients
4 cups (1L) fresh fruit, chopped
1/2 cup (125 mL) manuka honey
1/2 cup (125 mL) water or 1/2 cup (125 mL) yogurt
4 Tbsp (60 mL) spirulina or chlorella powder (optional)

Instructions
In a food processor, blend 3 cups of fruit and all other ingredients until just smooth. Pour into single-portion freezable containers. Popsicle containers are great for kids and all ages who are young at heart! Finish by inserting the remainder of the fresh fruit into the containers prior to freezing. Makes 4-5 cups (1-1.25L) of smoothie liquid.

Apple Crisp

Ingredients
Filling
10-12 large cooking apples, peeled and sliced (if you're in a hurry, leave the peels on)
Juice of one medium lemon
1/2 cup (125 mL) chopped fresh or frozen cranberries
1 tsp (5 mL) cinnamon

Topping
2 cups (500 mL) raw oats
1/2 cup (125 mL) whole wheat flour
1 tsp (5 mL) cinnamon
1/2 tsp (1 mL) nutmeg
1/4 cup (60 mL) sweetened coconut
2 Tbsp (30 mL) flaxseed meal
1/4 cup (60 mL) chopped nuts (pecans are great!)
1/2 cup (125 mL) honey or real maple syrup
1 cup apple juice (not from concentrate, to be poured over apples and topping)

Instructions
Preheat oven to 350°F (180°C). Mix together apples, lemon juice, cranberries, and cinnamon. Put apple mixture into a deep 8 in x 8 in (20 cm x 20 cm) casserole dish. Mix topping ingredients until well blended and spread on top of filling. Pour apple juice over entire mixture and bake uncovered until apples are soft, for about 45-60 minutes. A mixture of apples, berries, pears, or peaches makes a very special variation for the filling. Makes 6 servings.

Blueberry Muffins

Ingredients
3/4 cup (180 mL) rice milk
1 cup (250 mL) oatmeal
1 cup (250 mL) whole-wheat flour
1 tsp (5 mL) non-alum baking powder
1/2 tsp (2 mL) baking soda
1/4 tsp (1 mL) sea salt
1 cup (250 mL) organic blueberries
1 free-range egg or Flax Egg Replacer (see page 163)
1/4 cup (60 mL) melted coconut butter
1/3 cup (80 mL) honey

Instructions
Preheat oven to 400°F (200°C). In a medium bowl, combine rice milk and oatmeal; soak for 10 minutes. Combine flour, baking powder, baking soda, and sea salt in a separate bowl. Fold in blueberries.

Beat egg lightly in a medium bowl. Add melted coconut butter and honey to egg and beat. Blend together egg mixture and oatmeal.

Add moist mixture to dry blueberry mixture and stir lightly. Fill a muffin tray with paper muffin liners. Fill them to the top. Bake for 20 minutes or until a toothpick comes out clean. Makes 12 muffins.

Snicker Snacker Instant Treats

Create your own variations of this recipe by using whatever ingredients you have handy. Substitute ground pumpkin seeds, almonds, cashews, finely chopped dates, or raisins. A drop of vanilla or a pinch of cinnamon will give these treats a new twist. Choose seeds and nuts that are organic, raw, unsalted, and unroasted.

Ingredients
1/2 cup (125 mL) sunflower seeds*
1/2 cup (125 mL) sesame seeds*
1/3-1/2 cup (80-125 mL) honey
1/2 cup (125 mL) nut butter (cashew, pumpkin, peanut, or a mixture of several)
1/2 cup (125 mL) unsweetened carob powder
1/4 cup (60 mL) flax meal, wheat germ, or oat bran
1/4 cup (60 mL) unsweetened coconut

*If you're feeding these to toddlers and you don't have a food processor, grind the seeds first in your coffee grinder.

Instructions
Add the ingredients one at a time and blend in a food processor until the mixture forms a ball. Pinch off small amounts and form into bite-size balls. For a special effect, roll the balls in extra sesame seeds or coconut. Store in an airtight container and refrigerate. Makes 24 bite-size balls.

Almond Butter Cookies

Ingredients
3/4 cup (175 mL) organic applesauce
3/4 cup (175 mL) honey
1/4 cup (60 mL) cold-pressed safflower or sunflower oil
1 medium banana
1 cup (250 mL) almond butter
3 cups (750 mL) whole wheat flour
1/2 tsp (2 mL) sea salt
2 tsp (10 mL) baking soda
1/3 cup (80 mL) cornstarch
1/2 cup (125 mL) raw almond pieces
Optional: Replace almond pieces with dried apricot or
        cranberry chunks.

Instructions
Blend applesauce, honey, oil, and banana in a food processor until smooth. In a large bowl, mix together almond butter, flour and salt. Add blended ingredients to the bowl, then add baking soda, cornstarch, and almond pieces.

Onto an ungreased cookie sheet, scoop rounded mounds of cookie dough, shaping and pressing with a fork. They should be about 1/2 inch thick and flat on top. Bake at 325°F (160°C) for 10-15 minutes until top and edges are light-medium brown. Makes 4 dozen cookies. They freeze well.

Spreads & Egg Replacement

Better Butter

Ingredients
1 (0.5 kg) pound butter
1 cup (250 mL) high-quality essential fatty-acid-rich oil (such as flaxseed oil, Udo's Choice oil, Omega's Essential Balance, or any other organic, cold-pressed oil)

Instructions
Cut butter into eight pieces. Put butter and oil into the food processor and blend until smooth. Spoon into a covered container and refrigerate. Not only will you have better butter, but it will remain soft even though refrigerated. Makes 2 cups (500 mL).

Coconut Butter-Flaxseed Spread

Ingredients
1/2 cup (125 mL) flaxseed oil
1 cup (250 mL) coconut butter

Instructions
Place flaxseed oil in freezer for 2 hours or more. Melt coconut butter on low temperature. Remove from heat. Add frozen flaxseed oil. Blend and keep in the fridge for up to six weeks. Store in an opaque container to prolong life. Don't use for cooking or baking. It can be used as a spread in place of butter and margarine. Makes 1 1/2 cups (375 mL).

Flax Egg Replacer

Ingredients
1 Tbsp (15 mL) flax powder
3 Tbsp (45 mL) water

Instructions
Put flax powder in a small bowl. Add water and mix. Let sit for 2-3 minutes. Use when thick. Can be used to replace one egg in recipes. Makes 1 egg replacement.

Mayonnaise

Ingredients
2 free-range egg yolks at room temperature
1/4 tsp (1 mL) dry mustard
1 tsp (5 mL) freshly squeezed lemon juice
1/4 tsp (1 mL) sea salt
1/2 cup (125 mL) cold-pressed sunflower seed oil
1/2 cup (125 mL) flaxseed oil, EFA-rich oil blend (e.g., Udo's Choice) or Omega's
    garlic-chili flaxseed oil

Instructions
Combine egg, mustard, lemon juice, and salt, and blend thoroughly in the food
processor. While the processor is still running, slowly add oils drop by drop. Mayonnaise
will slowly thicken. Adjust salt and lemon juice to taste.

Mayonnaise Variations
Many ingredients can be added to this mayonnaise recipe: Fresh, finely chopped herbs:
dill, parsley, tarragon, and basil work well. You can also add any or a combination of
the following:
1 tsp (5 mL) curry powder
1 puréed avocado
1 Tbsp (15 mL) puréed sun-dried tomatoes
1 Tbsp (15 mL) finely chopped green onion

Makes 1 cup (250 mL).

9. Heart-Healthy Nutrients

"Find the seed at the bottom of your heart and bring forth a flower."

— Shigenori Kameoka

Many nutritionists and dieticians advise that we can get adequate vitamins and minerals from the foods we eat. But "adequate" is just not good enough anymore — especially if we want to prevent or treat heart disease.

People often resist making diet changes or adding nutrients until a health crisis forces them to rethink what their body needs. In a perfect world, you could obtain all the nutrients you need from the foods you eat, but today most people are eating the "SAD" — the Standard American Diet. For example, how many people eat the 7 to 10 half-cup (875-1,250 mL) servings of vegetables and fruits needed just to get the minimum basic nutrients for adequate health? Over 80 percent of North Americans eat just two servings of vegetables per day — and one of these is French fries.

With our exposure to environmental pollutants, stress, aging, and illness, we need even more vitamins, minerals, fatty acids, and coenzymes to keep disease at bay. And that is why you are most likely reading this book — because you already have some heart disease risks.

Cardiovascular nutrient research is an exciting area of study. It involves excellent clinical human research to show how effective nutrients are at not only preventing heart disease, but also treating existing cardiovascular problems.

Today, there are dozens of nutrients on the market for heart disease. The following are key nutrients that have been chosen for their scientific validity, safety, and effectiveness.

Sytrinol Lowers Cholesterol and Triglycerides in 30 Days

Sytrinol is a safe, effective cholesterol- and triglyceride-lowering nutrient that works in 30 days. It is comprised of a patented blend of powerful antioxidants, including polymethoxylated flavones (PMFs) and a range of palm (alpha, delta, and gamma) tocotrienols. Studies have revealed that sytrinol is able to significantly lower total cholesterol, bad cholesterol (LDL), and triglycerides and CRP, the inflammatory marker. Better still, this proprietary ingredient has also been shown to increase good cholesterol (HDL) levels.

Sytrinol Keeps Arteries Clear

Polymethoxylated flavones (PMFs), one of the main active ingredients in sytrinol, are a group of compounds derived from the peels of citrus fruits. The two most common are tangeretin and nobiletin, which are extremely potent bioflavonoids. More than 25 years of documented research provides evidence that these particular bioflavonoids deliver heart health benefits.

Nobiletin and tangeretin help lower levels of bad LDL by blocking the enzymes in the liver responsible for the manufacture of bad LDL building blocks: apolipoprotein B and triglycerides. Apolipoprotein B is considered the primary building block of bad cholesterol, making up almost 90 per cent of LDL cholesterol. Interestingly, triglycerides, the main kind of fat in your body, are one of the key contributors to the formation of apolipoprotein B.

Sytrinol is also comprised of palm tocotrienols, which, like tocopherols, are members of the vitamin E family and are extracted from the fruit of the palm tree. The palm tocotrienols in sytrinol come from Malaysia, a world leader in palm fruit sustainable farming. Like vitamin E, palm tocotrienols control anti-inflammatory responses and degrade HMG-CoA reductase, a key enzyme in your body used by your liver to produce cholesterol. Besides reducing cholesterol, palm tocotrienols have also been shown to inhibit arterial plaque formation and reduce blood clumping (platelet aggregation).

Sytrinol Is a Powerful Antioxidant

Palm tocotrienols are also powerful antioxidants, known to possess antioxidant potential far greater than that shown by vitamin E itself. In human studies, it was observed that alpha tocotrienols decreased the oxidation of bad LDL. This is important because high levels of LDL are a risk factor in cardiovascular disease. The antioxidant properties of tocotrienols can minimize damage caused by these compounds while protecting cell membranes.

Clinical results have shown that sytrinol exerts effects very similar to cholesterol-lowering statin drugs but without side-effects.

Sytrinol Improves Your LDL:HDL Ratio

To date, three main studies have been carried out to investigate sytrinol's effects on high cholesterol levels. The first study involved 60 participants with raised cholesterol levels. After prescribing 300 mg of sytrinol each day for four weeks, researchers found that sytrinol lowered total cholesterol by 25 percent, the bad LDL cholesterol by 19 percent, and triglycerides by 24 percent.

In the second, smaller study, 10 subjects with elevated cholesterol levels benefited after four weeks of treatment with 300 mg of sytrinol per day. Sytrinol therapy lowered total cholesterol levels by 20 percent, LDL cholesterol by 22 percent, apolipoprotein B (a component of LDL) by 21 percent, and triglycerides by 28 percent. Participants also had a significant five percent increase in apolipoprotein A1, an important structural protein of the good HDL cholesterol.

Researchers have now completed a third clinical trial, a 12-week placebo-controlled study involving 120 men and women with moderately elevated cholesterol levels. Compared to those in the placebo group, subjects taking sytrinol had a 30 percent drop in total cholesterol, 27 percent in LDL cholesterol, and 34 percent in triglycerides. In addition, HDL levels increased by 4 percent, resulting in a significant 29 percent improvement in the LDL:HDL ratio.

The best news is that sytrinol worked independently of diet changes. Toxicity studies have shown that sytrinol is well tolerated, with no toxic effects following consumption of sytrinol equalling up to one percent of total dietary intake, or the equivalent of a 150-pound person consuming almost 14 grams per day — that is nearly 50 times the recommended daily dosage of sytrinol at 300 mg per day.

Four human clinical trials have demonstrated that sytrinol reduced total cholesterol by 30 percent, LDL cholesterol by 27 percent, and triglycerides by 34 percent when compared to placebo.

Sytrinol ® Blood Cholesterol Study

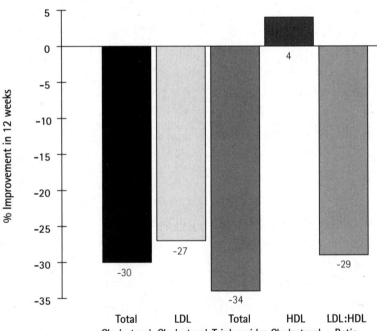

12-week placebo controlled/120 men & women
Reprinted with permission: KGK Synergize Inc.

Sytrinol's Five Actions Maintain a Healthy Heart

Total Cholesterol Benefits

Sytrinol's tocotrienols work by inhibiting the rate-limiting enzyme HMG-CoA reductase in the liver. However, sytrinol's mode of action contrasts with the competitive inhibition of HMG-CoA reductase receptors exhibited by statin drugs. The cholesterol-lowering effect of sytrinol appears to act by a novel process that controls the degradation rate of the HMG-CoA reductase enzyme. In other words, rather than actually preventing the manufacture of HMG-CoA reductase enzyme, which statin drugs do, the tocotrienols in sytrinol reduce the levels of this important enzyme required for cholesterol by increasing the rate at which the enzyme molecules degrade. As a result, sytrinol increases the rate of natural degradation of HMG-CoA reductase and reduces total cholesterol without the side-effects associated with statins.

LDL Benefits

Sytrinol's PMFs are known to reduce both apolipoprotein B levels needed for the manufacture of LDL particles and reduce levels of microsomal triglyceride transfer protein, which is needed to transfer fat into the bad LDL particles.

Triglyceride Benefits

PMFs are known to reduce DGAT activity (diacylglycerol acteyl transferase) and increase liver PPAR (peroxisome proliferator activated receptor). In doing so, PMFs reduce overall manufacture of triglyceride (DGAT inhibition) and increase fatty acid oxidation, thereby reducing triglyceride levels in the blood by two complementary mechanisms.

Anti-inflammatory Benefits

Inflammation, as we have learned, is a major trigger in heart disease. Studies are showing that heart disease is afflicting younger and younger people. One-third of those are in good health and their cholesterol is within normal ranges. Both men and women in this group have been shown to suffer from sudden heart attacks with no warning signs or risk factors known to cause heart disease. As you read earlier, recent research has established that inflammation may be the cause, as inflammation causes C-reactive protein (CRP), a known marker for sudden heart attack, to be produced in the body. Researchers have also shown that the presence of CRP in the body is a more reliable predictor of a pending heart attack than any other traditionally known risk factor for heart disease.

PMF's nobiletin and tangeretin have been studied for their anti-inflammatory properties, showing that the PMFs found in sytrinol would have a positive effect on CRP.

Antioxidant Benefits
PMFs and tocotrienols are among many natural potent antioxidants that have been researched for decades. PMFs can help protect blood vessel linings and prevent the oxidation of bad LDL cholesterol, which can lead to cardiovascular disease. Tocotrienols reduce oxidative damage, as well as the incidence of chronic diseases such as heart disease and cancer.

Muscle pain and weakness (myopathy) associated with statin use in 10 to 15 percent of patients has been considered a "minor" adverse affect. The extent to which these symptoms reflect underlying injury has been unknown; however, the results of a 2009 study in the *Canadian Medical Association Journal* by Swedish researchers found that persistent pain and weakness reflects "structural muscle damage" and that "alternative treatment strategies for patients with muscle symptoms need to be evaluated."

Sytrinol is not only advantageous compared to statin medications, but has also been shown to be a superior therapy in its ability to safely reduce cholesterol without side-effects, which even some natural remedies have. For example, red yeast rice, a common cholesterol-lowering natural remedy, is almost identical to prescription statins in

Statins: Expensive and Risky

Statins are the number-one-selling prescription drug in North America today. Statins are typically used to lower cholesterol and belong to a drug category known as HMG-CoA reductase inhibitors. Commonly used branded drugs in this category include: atorvastatin (Lipitor), cerivastatin (Baycol), lovastatin (Mevacor), pravastatin (Pravachol), rosuvastatin (Crestor) and simvastatin (Zocor). They are costly, and depending on dosage (the dosage range is 10-80 mg per day), their use is estimated to cost $3-8 per day or $90-240 per month.

Statins are typically prescribed with the goal of lowering LDL cholesterol. They work on inhibiting cholesterol manufacture and increasing the number of LDL receptors in the liver. Use of statins is not without risk, however. Some side-effects are:

- Muscle pain, weakness, and damage
- Nerve damage
- Measurable decline in cognition
- Increased risk of cancer
- Liver problems
- Joint pain
- Heart failure
- Muscle inflammation

Statins are disruptive to the natural overall balance of the body, blocking the natural production of coenzyme Q10, which shares the same metabolic pathway as statins (see page 175 for more information).

chemical structure and blocks the same pathway. Adding to consumer safety concerns, Consumer Labs reported that 40 percent of red yeast rice products tested in the U.S. contained toxic citrinin, and the amount of lovastatin (statin drug) in each product varied more than 100-fold. A UCLA study supports the Consumer Labs findings as it showed that only one of nine red yeast rice supplements bought in health food stores contained all the monacolins that lower cholesterol, and seven of nine red yeast rice supplements contained measurable concentrations of toxic citrinin. Canada has banned red yeast rice extracts. In the U.S., the FDA has taken the position that "red yeast rice products containing standardized lovastatin levels are unapproved new drugs." Clearly, red yeast rice has been, and continues to be, under heavy regulatory scrutiny, and safety concerns persist.

Sytrinol daily dose: 300 mg per day with or without food

Sytrinol should not be taken with sterols, another natural remedy for improving your lipid profile (triglycerides and cholesterol), because sterols inhibit sytrinol's absorption and reduce the effectiveness.

Pycnogenol Protects the Heart

Pycnogenol is standardized extract from the bark of the French maritime pine tree. The extract contains a potent blend of active phenolic compounds, including: catechin, taxifolium, procyanidins, and phenolic acids. Pycnogenol is known to be one of the most potent antioxidant compounds currently known. In fact, research has demonstrated that pycnogenol is up to 100 times more powerful than vitamin E. Pycnogenol is extremely effective at inactivating and neutralizing free radicals (molecules that damage any structure they contact). And pycnogenol has the ability to recycle and prolong the life span of key antioxidant vitamins C and E. Antioxidants protect against the cell-damaging effects of free radicals. Free radicals, as we learned earlier, are byproducts of normal physiological processes like digestion, for example, and their production can be exacerbated by lifestyle and environmental factors. Since free radicals are considered a major cause of aging and play a key role in the development of age-related diseases such as heart disease and dementia, the use of powerful antioxidants like pycnogenol may counteract some of the problems associated with aging.

♥ Pycnogenol helps:
- prevent blood clots
- protect DNA from damage
- lower blood sugar levels when elevated
- normalize high blood pressure
- reduce the risk of cancer
- protect cells from UV radiation damage
- protect against the damaging effects of cigarette smoke
- improve sperm quality
- improve wound healing
- improve lung function in asthmatics
- ease menstrual cramps

Pycnogenol Lowers High Blood Pressure

Research examining the effects of pycnogenol on high blood pressure showed it significantly lowered blood pressure in patients with moderately high blood pressure: 200 mg of pycnogenol daily was enough to dramatically reduce both systolic and diastolic blood pressure. It is believed that pycnogenol's ability to elevate nitric oxide production is the primary reason for reduced blood pressure. Nitric oxide causes blood vessels to relax, increasing blood flow and decreasing blood pressure.

Common Side-effects of Blood Pressure Lowering Drugs

- Depression
- Palpitations
- Constipation
- Impotence
- Kidney damage
- Rapid heart rate
- Insomnia

Pycnogenol — Blood Clot Preventer

Pycnogenol is also effective at reducing blood clots. Belcaro and researchers evaluated the risk of deep vein thrombosis (DVT) during flights longer than eight hours. Those participants using pycnogenol had no cases of deep vein thrombosis whereas, in the group taking a placebo, there were five cases of thrombosis. Like previous research, it is believed that pycnogenol's ability to relax blood vessels (which increases blood flow) is the reason for reduced blood clots. Other research has also shown that pycnogenol reduces the stickiness of blood. Reducing the risk of blood clots is particularly important since we know blood clots can cause strokes and heart attacks. Every 35 seconds in North America someone has a stroke.

Pycnogenol Repairs Capillaries

As we age, our blood vessels lose their elasticity and can leak. Pycnogenol repairs damaged blood vessels by enhancing collagen. Collagen is the component that makes our skin smooth and our nails, hair, and bones strong. It also provides shape and flexibility to our blood vessels, capillaries, and veins — all part of a healthy vascular system.

Pycnogenol Prevents Fat Deposition in Artery Walls

Fatty deposits in our arteries are a major factor in coronary artery disease. Pycnogenol can also help prevent the buildup of fatty deposits in artery walls. When LDL, the bad cholesterol, is oxidized, it becomes sticky and accumulates on the inner lining of blood vessels. Blood flow is reduced as the deposits become thicker. When this occurs to the capillaries supplying the heart, it can lead to a heart attack if blood supply is completely blocked. Pycnogenol was found to reduce the oxidation of LDL cholesterol and prevent the buildup of fatty deposits.

Pycnogenol daily dose: 30mg-200mg per day with meals

Coenzyme Q10 — The Heart Superstar

Coenzyme Q10 or ubiquinone, often referred to as CoQ10 or Q10, is one of the most powerful antioxidants known for helping maintain a healthy heart. Although CoQ10 has been described as a coenzyme, it functions more like a vitamin. Vitamins by definition are essential and coenzyme CoQ10 is a micronutrient that supports biochemical reactions in the body. Coenzyme Q10 is produced naturally by the body, but production declines as we age. By 50, everyone should be taking a daily supplement of CoQ10.

Coenzyme Q10 exists in the mitochondria, the powerhouse of our cells. CoQ10 enhances energy at the cellular level, especially in the heart, enabling your heart muscle to pump blood efficiently. With the help of CoQ10, ATP (adenosine triphosphate) is made inside the mitochondria and provides the fuel that gives the entire body energy. CoQ10 acts as the battery charger for the energy system in the heart and other body cells. The heart is one of the few organs that never takes a rest; it is continuously functioning. This is the main reason CoQ10 is probably the single best nutrient that you can take for a healthy heart.

Statin Drugs Deplete Q10

Statin drugs inhibit the body's manufacture of CoQ10 just like they do cholesterol, so the reduction of CoQ10 in the body when taking statins is not a side-effect but an inherent function of the statin drugs. Statin drugs can decrease the body's manufacture of CoQ10 by as much as 40 percent. It is imperative if you are taking statin drugs that you supplement with CoQ10 daily.

In 2007, the *American Journal of Cardiology* published a study of 32 patients with muscle symptoms associated with the use of statins. The patients were randomly divided into two groups. For one month, one group took daily CoQ10 at a dosage of 100 mg while the other took 400 IU (international units) of vitamin E daily. After 30 days, the patients who received CoQ10 experienced a 40 percent reduction in the severity of pain associated with statin use. No significant changes were found among those who received vitamin E.

♥ Multipurpose CoQ10

Not only does CoQ10 provide a strong, healthy heart, but it also helps:

• Maintain healthy cholesterol ratio

• Protect all cellular membranes

• Halt free radical damage because it is a powerful antioxidant

• Keep gums strong and prevents and treats gingivitis
 (a risk factor for cardiovascular disease)

• Support healthy skin

• Slow cellular aging

Statins Increase Breast Cancer Risk

Statin medication use is also associated with increased breast cancer risk. One study in the Procedures of the *American Society of Clinical Oncology* found that the incidence of breast cancer increases when women use statin medications. A total of 66,843 women over 35 were included in the study. Statin use was identified from pharmacy data collected from 1997 until 2002. Statins were found to increase estradiol levels in women. Estradiol is a strong estrogen associated with abnormal cell growth. The average age of women in the research group taking statins who developed breast cancer was 57.6 years. The researchers reported that women taking statin medications should be advised of the potential increased risk of breast cancer.

Dietary sources of CoQ10 include beef heart, pork and chicken liver, mackerel, sardines, walnuts, and strawberries, to name a few. Q10 is particularly concentrated in organ meats. With the recommendation that people reduce their consumption of red meat, a natural decline in our consumption of CoQ10 occurs as well. Nevertheless, well over 100 clinical studies at major health institutions have documented CoQ10's heart-protective abilities.

CoQ10 Lowers Blood Pressure

A meta-analysis of human clinical trials using CoQ10 for high blood pressure was led by Professor Frank Rosenfeldt, Director of the Cardiac Surgical Research Unit at Alfred Hospital in Melbourne, Australia. His team reviewed all published trials of CoQ10 for hypertension and assessed overall efficacy, consistency of therapeutic action, and side-effect incidence. The meta-analysis evaluated 12 clinical trials involving 362 patients comprising three randomized controlled trials, one crossover study, and eight open-label studies. The Australian group concluded that coenzyme Q10 has the potential in hypertensive patients to lower systolic blood pressure by up to 17 mmHg and diastolic blood pressure by up to 10 mmHg without significant side-effects.

Cardiovascular Benefits of CoQ10

Congestive Heart Failure

CoQ10 in conjunction with standard treatments dramatically improves outcomes in clinical studies of congestive heart failure, which is classified as impairment of the heart's ability to pump enough blood for all the body's needs. Doses of 300 mg per day have been shown to improve the heart's ability to pump in those with congestive heart failure. CoQ10's antioxidant activity may also contribute to its benefits in treating congestive heart failure.

Stable Angina

CoQ10 has been studied in humans for stable angina since the early 1980s. Angina patients taking 150 mg per day of CoQ10 report a greater ability to exercise without the onset of angina. CoQ10 is also clinically demonstrated to substantially improve arrythmias and hypertension.

♥ Baby Aspirin or Ginger?

Aspirin, with its blood-thinning and anti-inflammatory properties, is often recommended to reduce the risk of heart attack reoccurrence. People concerned with heart disease risk are also often counseled to take aspirin preventatively. However, blanket recommendations on the latter point are something the U.S. Preventive Services Task Force attempted to avoid in its 2002 official opinion on aspirin. Given knowledge that aspirin increases the incidence of gastrointestinal bleeding and some evidence that aspirin increases incidence of hemorrhagic stroke, the Task Force suggested that doctors discuss aspirin use only with patients found to be at high risk of heart disease (those with a 10-year risk of at least six percent).

A May 2002 article in *The New England Journal of Medicine* took a more moderate stance against aspirin use by concluding that those with a 10-year risk of 15 percent are good candidates for aspirin treatment. Clearly, aspirin use in heart disease is not a cut-and-dried situation. Research continues. Women over 70 should avoid aspirin as it can increase the risk of stroke. For those who have had a heart attack, angioplasty, or bypass surgery, a baby aspirin a day can be taken if advised by your physician. However, gastrointestinal bleeding is a common side-effect of even a baby aspirin per day. In January 2009, the *International Journal of Cardiology* stated that ginger is an effective anti-platelet herb. Drink ginger tea daily, use grated ginger on foods, and take ginger capsules as an alternative to baby aspirin.

Bad Cholesterol Oxidation

As mentioned earlier, oxidation of LDL cholesterol in the blood is a key factor in development of cardiovascular disease, and CoQ10 prevents this even more effectively than vitamin E. CoQ10 has also been shown to help reduce the adverse side-effects of cardiotoxic chemotherapy drugs, including adriamycin and athralines.

Coenzyme Q10 daily dose: Maintenance dose: 30-100 mg per day with food. Those with congestive heart failure should take 300 mg/day. If using statin medications, you need 100-200 mg/day. Those with high blood pressure should take 100-200 mg per day.

Marvelous Magnesium

Although magnesium is responsible for over 350 enzymatic functions in the human body, its major role is in the overall health of the heart. As mentioned in Chapter 6, magnesium is likened to "nature's calcium channel-blocker" because of its ability to block the entry of calcium into vascular smooth-muscle cells and heart muscle cells. As a result, in addition to eating high-magnesium foods, magnesium supplementation can help lower blood pressure, improve vascular function, and aid efficient heart function. Magnesium also helps regulate proper calcium metabolism by acting on several hormones, including parathyroid hormone and calcitonin in the thyroid.

Potassium and Sodium Need Magnesium

Without magnesium, potassium and sodium cannot be pumped into and out of cells. So magnesium deficiency is often the culprit when potassium deficiency is suspected. If you have added potassium to your diet, and still have not seen an improvement in heart health, it may be because the potassium is not getting inside the cells where it is needed due to lack of magnesium.

Magnesium Protects Against Stroke

In one study, 14,221 men and women aged 45–64 provided blood samples to measure their magnesium levels. Over the course of 15 years of follow-up, researchers found that blood levels of magnesium were significantly associated with decreased risks of stroke. Specifically, participants taking over 270 mg per day had a 30 percent decreased risk of stroke.

Researchers attributed magnesium's effect on stroke risk reduction on its ability to help maintain healthy blood pressure and to help maintain blood sugar health. Magnesium deficiency is associated with increased inflammation, which increases circulating levels of CRP, which triggers cell damage in blood vessel cells.

Not All Magnesium Supplements are Created Equal

Magnesium supplements are available in numerous salt forms (e.g., magnesium oxide, gluconate, chloride), and are also bound to amino acids. The absorption rate and tolerability varies greatly between different magnesium supplements. Many are poorly tolerated at therapeutic doses due to magnesium's laxative effect.

Magnesium in its inorganic state (simple salt) is only absorbed at 5 to 10 percent. Inorganic minerals must be altered from their natural state before they can penetrate the intestinal barrier. The most efficient way to achieve this is by combining them with amino acids. Magnesium joined to the amino acid glycine is the best form because it is best absorbed by the body and also able to cross the blood-brain barrier.

Magnesium Lowers Bad Cholesterol
While Increasing Good

Magnesium works its magic on cholesterol in two ways. One, it regulates enzymes that control the production of cholesterol. Second, it increases levels of good cholesterol while lowering bad cholesterol. Dr. Mildred Seelig, the famous magnesium researcher, concludes that Lipitor works by inhibiting the production of the HMG Coenzyme A reductase enzyme that is produced by the liver. This enzyme is also necessary for the production of coenzyme Q10, which is critical for optimal heart health. HMG Coenzyme A reductase is also converted into another compound known as mevalonate, a fatty acid derivative. Mevalonate is also converted into cholesterol or it can be converted into several plaque-forming substances. Dr. Seelig found that as long as the body has adequate magnesium, it will naturally regulate the HMG Coenzyme

A and cholesterol manufacture will be controlled. But if you become deficient in magnesium, the HMG Coenzyme A will increase plaque formation in the arteries. Magnesium is key to keeping arteries clear and cholesterol levels healthy.

Magnesium Regulates Blood Pressure

Magnesium supplements have a significant effect on lowering high blood pressure. But some research results have indicated that magnesium lowered high blood pressure whereas other research did not. Now, Japanese researchers have finally clarified inconsistent results from other magnesium/high blood pressure investigations. They followed individuals over an eight-week period. The results showed that blood pressure was significantly lowered while taking magnesium. And the higher the blood pressure, the larger the decrease seen in those supplementing with magnesium. Researchers believe magnesium acts to relax blood vessels, an effect proven to help lower blood pressure. When blood vessels are constricted — not relaxed — the heart works harder to pump blood through the body, causing blood pressure to increase.

Women should be particularly interested in magnesium supplementation if they have high blood pressure. Often, traditional high blood pressure medications do not work as well for women, but magnesium supplementation works fabulously in women to normalize high blood pressure. However, high blood pressure medications can cause erectile dysfunction in men. With this in mind, men should be employing natural remedies to reduce high blood pressure as well.

Magnesium glycinate daily dose: 280-500 mg with food

Multivitamins and Minerals to the Rescue

A good multivitamin with minerals is important for preventing heart problems. Multivitamins with minerals contain potassium along with other necessary cofactors for a healthy heart, including B vitamin complex, beta-carotene, vitamins A, C, E, as well as the minerals selenium, magnesium, and calcium.

Vitamin E improves circulation, has natural gentle blood-thinning properties, reduces oxidized bad cholesterol, and helps prevent heart disease. In a multivitamin with mineral formula, look for a dosage of 200 IU of natural (d-alpha-tocopherol) vitamin E per day. If you are on Coumadin or Warfarin, you can take 200 IU per day but not more.

Two types of vitamin A are available: preformed vitamin A, or retinols, and precursor vitamin A, known as beta-carotene and sourced from plants. Beta-carotene is converted into vitamin A in the body. Stored in the liver and fat soluble, beta carotene in dosages of 12,500 IU per day has been shown to protect the heart. Several controversial studies using extremely high doses of beta carotene and vitamin A — 75,000 IU per day — found it caused adverse effects.

B vitamins and folic acid have been found to lower the risk of heart disease and heart attack. High homocysteine is a risk factor for heart disease because it can cause cholesterol to create plaque formation on the walls of arteries and vessels. B vitamins, especially B5, B3, B12, and folic acid, can help reduce homocysteine.

Vitamin C, a potent antioxidant, protects blood vessel linings and lowers lipoprotein A (Lp(a)), a type of cholesterol linked to increased risk of heart disease.

It is easier to get these nutrients in a good multivitamin with minerals. Vitamins and minerals are the foundation of your heart health nutrient program. A recent study into the use of vitamins in relation to mortality found that multivitamins and vitamin E were associated with decreased risks of cardiovascular disease mortality. Always take your multi-nutrient formula with food.

♥ What Makes a Great Multivitamin with Minerals?

Scientists at Harvard Medical School have advised all adults to take multivitamins with minerals every day to help prevent deficiencies of nutrients that may contribute to a multitude of health problems. Suboptimal levels of folic acid and vitamins B6 and B12, deficient levels of calcium and vitamin D, can all contribute to degenerative disease.

While the market is flooded with multi-nutrient formulas, many contain only the Food and Drug Administration's or Health Canada's recommended dietary allowance (RDAs) of vitamins and minerals. While those amounts may be sufficient to prevent diseases such as scurvy, we know that heart health requires nutrients in optimal amounts.

Research also shows that the body more readily uses certain forms of vitamins and minerals than others. Many vitamin combinations on the market today use the cheapest, least absorbable forms of vitamins and minerals available or, worse yet, do not label what forms are found in the pill. Make sure you purchase nutrients from a reputable company that manufactures under good manufacturing processes (GMP). Also make sure that a third party independently tests the finished nutrients for potency and purity. And further make sure the label states the type of nutrient and the quality. Your multi-nutrient formula should disclose the source of its ingredients. For example, instead of just saying magnesium, the label should say magnesium (as citrate, oxide, chelate, or glycinate).

Is your multi-nutrient formula in capsule form? Most people find capsules easier to digest. The formula should also be designed for your unique needs. If you are a woman, you will need different nutrients than a man.

Niacin — Proven Cholesterol-busting Vitamin

Researchers at the University of Pennsylvania Medical Center stated that niacin or nicotinic acid, a water-soluble B vitamin, is the oldest and least used, least expensive method to significantly lower cholesterol. Niacin reduces LDL-cholesterol levels by 10-20 percent, reduces triglycerides by 20-50 percent, and raises HDL-cholesterol by 15-35 percent. A randomized, controlled comparison of the cholesterol-lowering statin drug lovastatin (Mevacor) found that niacin lowers LDL (bad cholesterol) to a similar degree (23 percent [niacin] vs. 32 percent [statin]), while elevating HDL considerably more (33 vs. 6 percent). Niacin also lowers lipoprotein(a) (Lp(a)) by an astounding 35 percent while lovastatin therapy has no effect.

Niacin has a common, harmless side-effect of skin flushing that is caused by the dilation of blood vessels. Over time, after building a tolerance to niacin, this flushing is reduced or stops altogether. Nicotinamide or niacinamide, another form of niacin, does not lower cholesterol levels and should not be used in place of niacin. Niacin in doses high enough to alter cholesterol levels can have side-effects including elevated liver enzymes, and is not recommended for those with gout. Because of the potential side-effects of regular niacin, it is recommended that you use the non-flushing form of niacin called inositol hexanicotinate (also known as inositol niacinate), which is side-effect free. Researchers have found non-flushing niacin to be more effective than niacin in its cholesterol-lowering, blood-pressure-lowering, and lipotropic (fat-metabolizing) effects. This form of niacin is slowly metabolized in the body.

Non-flushing Niacin for Intermittent Claudication
Inositol hexanicotinate has also been used to improve blood flow in the treatment of intermittent claudication (a painful cramp in calf muscles produced by a decreased oxygen supply to the muscles). Some studies show that compared to niacin, inositol hexanicotinate is safer and better tolerated.

Non-flushing Niacin Lowers Fibrinogen
Fibrinogen, a protein produced in the liver, is a necessary part of the normal blood-clotting process. But when fibrinogen levels get too high — as can happen in conditions of inflammation — fibrinogen can increase your odds of forming dangerous blood clots, which can plug off a blood vessel leading into your heart, triggering a heart attack. Fibrinogen also causes

smooth muscle cells to multiply, which can promote atherosclerosis. People whose fibrinogen levels are high have roughly double the risk of heart disease than people with low fibrinogen levels.

Niacin daily dose: 1,500 mg at breakfast and 1,500 mg at bedtime

Heart Health Nutrient Program

Nutrient	Daily dose
Sytrinol	300 mg with or without food
Pycnogenol	30-200 mg with food
Coenzyme Q10	30-300 mg with food
Magnesium	280-500 mg with food
Non-flushing niacin	1,500 mg at breakfast, 1,500 mg at bedtime
Echium oil	1-2 tsp (5-10 mL) with food
Selenomethionine	100 mcg with food
Vitamin K2 MK7	100 mcg with food
Multivitamin with minerals	As directed

10. Heart Health Fitness Training

"What the heart knows today,
the head will understand tomorrow."

— James Stephens

If you asked 100 people what the optimal activity for cardiovascular health was, the bulk of them would probably answer, "aerobic activity." While it is indeed crucial for the heart muscle, a weight program, in fact, is also a pivotal part of a healthy-heart lifestyle. In this chapter, we will tell you why and teach you how to begin your weight-training program properly, the equipment you'll need, and the cutting-edge core training information you can use for optimal physical performance during your routine. Finally, you will uncover a specialized time-saving, 20-minute exercise weight-training and cardio program spaced out over 10 days that can be repeated indefinitely to help you attain total heart health and vitality.

Weights: Invaluable for Heart Health

Almost everyone is aware that a walk around the block, a light jog through the neighborhood woods or playing sports, and just generally getting out there and doing something is the key for a healthier ticker. So, the obvious question you might be asking yourself right now is: Why would you need to do weights to keep your heart healthy?

First, you need muscle to do every physical activity on earth, even if it is just for going for a walk around the block. It takes about 276 muscles coordinating together just to take a single step, so you can be sure your need for muscle is very real and very important to your well-being. More specifically, it is invaluable to your long-term well-being. And remember, as you age, your muscle starts to disappear. Poor muscle tone causes additional stress on the heart as you struggle to perform daily tasks.

♥ Four Tips Before You Begin

See a doctor. Before you begin any exercise and/or diet program, you should definitely get medical clearance to ensure your personal safety and well-being.

Breathe. Be sure to breathe during any physical activity you enjoy, including your resistance workout. We have a natural tendency to hold our breath to create additional internal pressure to aid us in resisted movements. However, though holding our breath may give us the feeling of additional strength, it does not bode well for our internal circulatory system. In fact, it puts undue pressure on your entire circulatory system, including your heart, so do not ever hold your breath during any part of your exercise program, even if it is just for a split second.

Start at your level. Many programs start everyone at the same level. Since we are all different, you should try to start at a level that gives you a good workout without leaving you too tired or wanting more. For example, if you begin this program and find that one or two of the exercises are too easy, do not be afraid to add a couple extra reps or use 5 to 10 percent heavier resistance. This does not mean trying to do an exercise with poor form; it means upgrading when you are completely proficient at an exercise. Upgrading will help insure you do not plateau and, after you have found your starting point for each exercise, you will probably find it takes a minimum of three to five weeks to become proficient at a given exercise before it is time to upgrade it again. You can upgrade by adding up to 20 reps total per exercise, or you can begin using heavier dumbbells.

Take breaks. If you need a break during the program or if you need to take a day off because of fatigue or sickness, take it. Listen to your body and give it the extra time to recover if it needs to, and you will actually see faster and better results.

That is why weight training needs to be part of this equation because it will allow you to build and maintain more muscle on your frame, which will translate into your having more muscle down the road to do the activities that will keep you younger for longer. This will help nullify the "muscle loss effects" of aging. You will be able to do cardiovascular activities like sports and walking around the block more frequently and for greater duration, effectively keeping your heart healthier for more years than those who do not employ some form of resistance training. And if you do it, the muscle will stay on your frame. It is that simple.

Your heart is the most important muscle in your body, always working, 24-7, and if you exercise it appropriately, it will stay strong and healthy for years to come. Every other of the 616-odd muscles in your body responds in pretty much the same manner. If you use it, you will not lose it. Training, strengthening, and preserving your muscles will allow you to engage in vital heart health boosting exercises and daily activities well into your later years.

In fact, many of today's top health and fitness gurus are beginning to say that your muscular age is in fact indicative of your real age and not your chronological age. In other words, if you move and have more muscle and less fat, like a younger and healthier person would, then you actually are likely physiologically younger and healthier than someone who does not. So how do you wind back the clock and maintain a younger more youthful, heart healthy you? Start a resistance training program.

Here's the second benefit of weight training for heart health: All the lean muscle that weight training builds also means more calories burned and less fat stored on your waistline and along your artery walls.

Most current literature states that adding just one single pound of muscle to your physique can burn up to 50 extra calories a day! Adding just five pounds of muscle to your frame (which equals 50 extra calories burned per day) would be enough active tissue to burn just over 25 pounds of extra fat off you (or keep 25 pounds off you and out of your heart) over the next year. Factor in the osteoporosis-slowing and posture-improving effects of additional lean tissue and there are plenty of reasons to start a weight training program right away. Here is what you need to do before you start.

Why Walking Works

The human body is designed to walk. What better way to spend a sunny afternoon than to get outdoors, getting an aerobic workout, increasing our heart rate, increasing circulation, strengthening the heart muscle, filling our lungs with fresh air, and reaping the benefits of all that oxygen? A little rain never hurt anyone, either. What has really hurt many heart disease sufferers — and people with heart disease risk factors — is a sedentary lifestyle.

The benefits of walking for the heart are numerous. Moderate physical activity, including walking, cycling, and light gardening, for 30 minutes a day, cuts the risk of heart disease mortality. Even 35 minutes of exercise three times a week can reduce cardiovascular risks, as well as depression and emotional stress, better than conventional care alone.

Best of all, it is never too late to get strolling. A 2006 study in *Heart* reported that couch potatoes who only started exercising later in life still significantly cut their chances of developing heart disease. People aged 40-plus who got off that couch and got active lowered their risk by 55 percent compared to the still inactive. People who had been active and stayed active enjoyed a 60 percent drop in risk for coronary heart disease. In 2006, researchers also reviewed all the current literature on walking for the prevention of heart disease and its risk factors. They noted in the *Journal of Women's Health* that walking cuts a woman's risk and has beneficial effects on risk factors such as obesity, abnormal cholesterol and triglyceride levels, hypertension, and diabetes.

Equipment

Many of the exercises in this program make use of a set of dumbbells. Dumbbells can be purchased at your local department store for minimal cost. When choosing a set of dumbbells, pick a weight with which you can perform a bicep curl no more than 12 times and no less than 10. For most women, this weight will be between 8 to 12 pounds. Fifteen- to twenty-five-pound dumbbells will be sufficient for most men. Learning a bit of core training (see tips below) will make your dumbbells even more effective.

Easy Walking Tips

- Join a walking group. Starting and sticking to a fitness routine is easier if you are not alone.
- Walk during work. Skip the coffee break and head outside for 15 minutes of fresh air. The amount of cardiovascular exercise you do over a day adds up. You do not have to do 45 minutes in one session. Every 15 minutes counts.
- In bad weather, walk in a nearby shopping mall. Not only will you get a weather-proof workout, but you may find a great pair of shoes, too.
- Buy a pedometer. Set an initial, reasonable goal for yourself, e.g., 2,500 steps a day, and increase it as you achieve it.
- Schedule walks. Write them into your day-timer as you would any function or meeting. If the walk is at work, what better time to brainstorm than when the blood is pumping?
- Take your pet for a walk. A pet's squiggling enthusiasm is nothing but infectious.
- Take your family for a walk. They may not be quite as excited as your dog, but you do not have to pick up their poo, either.

Core Training Tips for Your Program

Your core muscles should be engaged during any and all of your physical activities. Whether it is gardening, a walk or jog around the block, or a toning and tightening workout with the weights, having your core muscles properly engaged will protect your spine, tone your abdominals quicker and enhance your overall posture. Here are some quick tips on basic core training.

- Your core is the abdominal musculature on your torso that links your upper body and lower body together. This torso area is also often thought of as your foundation.
- You can train it anytime and pretty much anywhere.
- The key to training your core is to have it engaged during exercise and other daily activities, so it supports the spine and strengthens and tightens the abdominal musculature.

- The main core muscles we are going to focus on are your transverse abdominis (TVA) and your kegels or pelvis floor muscles (these are the muscles used to stop the flow of urine).
- You fire up your TVA by drawing in your stomach toward your spine. You fire up your kegels by flexing the same way you would to stop the flow of urine. Flexing these muscles will engage your core and make it feel like there is more muscle tension in your deep lower abdominals and pelvic area.
- Here is another way to think of it: The core trick to tightening your tummy instantly, increasing your posture, and improving breathing and circulation is to: "Draw in your bikini bottom."

The key to targeting your core is to target it down low. Focus on drawing in your lower tummy, i.e., the part covered by your bikini bottom. Think of the center of the top edge of your bikini bottom as the center of your core (mark it in your mind with a red dot). Try to draw in that red dot. It is that easy: If you pull this area in, you will tighten your abdominal wall, thinning your waist and flattening out your tummy!

Core specialist and author Paul Chek states in his book *Eat, Move and Be Healthy* that: "The deep abdominal wall (TVA) is ideally suited to perform girdle-like supportive functions that allow you to have a flat stomach. The dreaded paunch belly is but one of the many ill effects of a dysfunctional wall." TVA is the key core muscle you engage to support your back and get you a flat stomach. Try this technique during all your exercises and other activities, even while driving, gardening, or sitting at the dinner table.

Though keeping your core engaged may make it slightly more difficult to breath, just be sure to maintain continuous breathing and, over time, you'll find it becomes less challenging to breath with your core engaged. Also, make sure you are not drawing your stomach in and "up" too much (this may be compressing your diaphragm slightly, making breathing a bit more difficult).

Notice that, with the core engaged, the back flattens out slightly. This is the basic position you should be looking for during most exercises. Conversely, try to avoid a swayback position or an overly flat back position for the safety of your back.

Now that you are primed and prepped with starter tips, equipment, and core training protocol, let's get you started on your program.

Program Outline

To save time and increase the benefit of every resistance exercise in this program, many of the exercises are combination exercises that will amalgamate two classic exercises. The first exercise on Day 1, for example, combines a squat with a bicep curl. These exercises will save time, add vital heart-helping muscle to your body, and boost your cardiovascular fitness much faster than would a single joint exercise, such as bicep curls. Each day finishes with a cardiovascular fitness option. You can personally choose from the list provided below to perform for 10 minutes or more at the end of each daily resistance training session. This combination of weights and cardiovascular exercise is the most optimal format for maximizing muscular and cardiovascular development. Below are a few more quick tips before we begin.

In summary: Each day, complete the warm-up described below, then complete the two exercises for each day and one of the cardio examples of your choice. Try to do a minimum of 5 to 10 minutes or more of cardio a day and, yes, you can repeat and or mix cardio activities over and over as many times as you like. In total, each day can be completed in as little as 10 to 15 minutes!

All sets of one exercise can be completed at once, or you can alternate between sets of the two exercises to save time. For example, you could complete three sets of squats, resting between each set of squats, and then move on to three sets of the next exercise. You then finish with your cardio. Or you could complete one set of squats, and then complete one set of the next exercise before returning to complete your second set of squats, and maintain said pattern until you finish all sets of both exercises. You would then finish with your cardio. Whichever format you choose, make sure you warm up before each training session so your body is ready for anything you throw at it.

Warm-up (every day)

Perform a light walk for five minutes on the treadmill with arm swings and side-to-side torso twists to get blood to all parts of the body and the synovial fluid (joint fluid) to the joints without high impact on the joints. Jogging on the spot for two to four minutes would also achieve the same effect if there is not an exercise machine nearby.

Make sure you complete this warm-up before every single workout or physical activity you perform. A proper warm-up is vital to maintaining the longevity of your joints and helping you get your heart rate up in a smooth, moderate fashion so it is primed for activity. Once you have completed this warm-up, ease into your first exercise slowly, then speed things up within your comfort zone as your routine unfolds. After that, top it off with some cardio from the list below to complete each day.

♥ Cardio Option List

(Choose one for each day and perform for 5 to 10 minutes or more after the two weight exercises)

Jogging on the spot, performing variations of butt kicks, high knees, jumping jacks, or other light-impact motions

Skipping	Cross-country skiing
Rebounding	Treadmill
Bicycling	Rowing
Swimming	Sports
Brisk walking	Landscaping, including cutting the lawn

Day 1

Exercise 1

Free Squat with Bicep Curl (add optional calf raises)

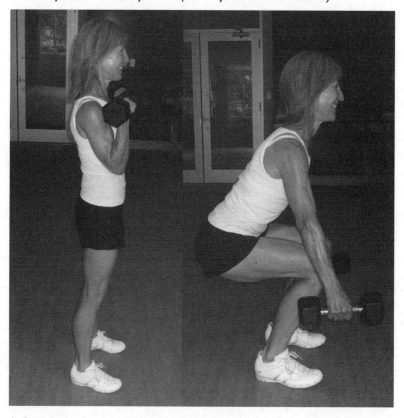

A free squat is the marquee total body exercise. It covers all of our major muscle groups to help support all our daily activities. It should be a staple of everyone's weight training program. Learning how to do a proper squat will benefit you every time you need to bend down, lift something, or strengthen and tone your body. This exercise is also going to burn a large number of calories and improve your cardiovascular endurance.

Begin by standing with your weights at your side, feet shoulder width apart. Start by driving your hips back as if you are trying to stick your butt out while letting your weights glide down to just outside your knee level. Maintain a "ski jump" curve in your lower back as you squat down to protect it from injury. From this bottom position, ascend up out of the squat, breathe out and complete your bicep curl.

Targets: Quads, Glutes, Biceps
Complete: 3 Sets of 12 to 15 Reps

Exercise 2
Dips with Hip Lifts on: Bench/Stairs/Coffee table

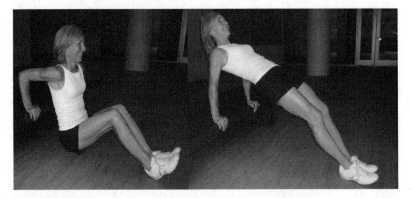

Beginner: 2 legs   Advanced: 1 leg
This is a challenging exercise. You may only be able to do a few short motion repetitions of it when you start out, which is fine. Stick with it and you will tighten and tone the triceps (backs of your upper arms) and your glutes and the backs of your thighs as well. This exercise targets three trouble spots at once and, with all this muscle working, it certainly qualifies as an exercise that will keep you moving and your heart pumping.

Begin by placing your hands at your sides with your fingers gripping the edge of your chosen apparatus. Your legs should be comfortably bent out in front of you. Drop your hips down and perform a dip to a depth you are comfortable with, then drive up with your arms until they lock out while pushing your hips up as high as you can.

* You can make this exercise easier or harder by bending or extending your legs to fit your fitness level.

Targets: Glutes, Hamstrings, Triceps
Complete: 3 Sets of 10 to 12 Reps

Exercise 3
Perform cardio option from list above for 5 to 10 minutes or more.

Day 2
Exercise 1
Squat "Ski Slope" Rows

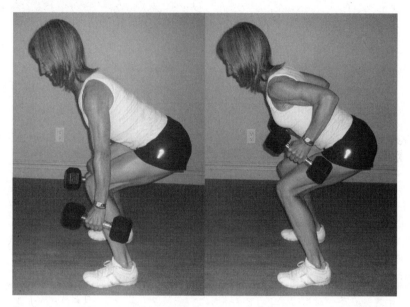

Every time you sit down to perform an exercise, you shut off around 70 percent or more of your muscle, so we are going to try and avoid doing so with as many exercises as possible. Instead of performing a classical "seated row," we are going to show you how to do a more challenging, yet far more beneficial, squat row.

Begin by performing the same squat you use with the "Free Squat with Bicep Curl" exercise on Day 1, and drop down to the bottom of the squat with your weights at your side. While maintaining your ski slope back position, pull the weights up to the sides of your ribcage and squeeze your shoulder blades together, then lower the weights down again and repeat.

Targets: Entire Back, Quads, Biceps
Complete: 3 Sets of 12 to 15 Reps

Exercise 2
Push-ups

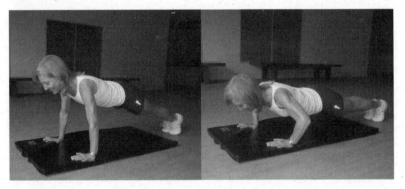

Yes, they are hard. Yes, they are tough and, yes, they might not be your favorite exercise, but they are one of the best upper body exercises of all time — especially for women! The benefits of push-ups far outweigh the challenges they present. That is why we are taking advantage of everything they do for our health and fitness.

Push-ups strengthen the major upper body muscles you use most in your daily life. In fact, push-ups work so much muscle that you get a great calorie burn, metabolism boost, and cardio hit from them.

If a full push-up is too difficult, begin with a push-up from your knees with your hands slightly wider than shoulder width apart and in line with your chest (make sure to put a pillow or pad beneath your knees even if you are on carpet). Drop down until your arms are at a 90-degree angle, then press up and squeeze your chest together at the top of each repetition.

Targets: Chest, Triceps, Core
Complete: 3 Sets of as many as you can do

Exercise 3

Perform cardio option from list above for 5 to 10 minutes or more.

Commute to Work – Your Heart Will Thank You

Are you thinking of walking or biking to work? Maybe you should. Active commuters have fewer heart disease risk factors than non-commuters, says a new 2009 report in the *Archives of Internal Medicine*. Men and women who walk and ride to work are fitter, leaner, have healthier triglyceride and blood sugar levels, and better blood pressure, indicating that this form of "lifestyle exercise," as it has been branded, is beneficial in the fight against heart disease. The added bonus is that walking and riding are better for the environment, too.

Day 3
Exercise 1
Step Back Lunge with Bicep Curl

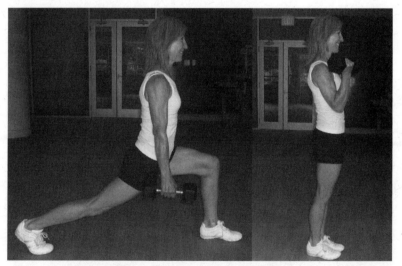

Lunges are another great classic exercise. They burn lots of calories and target tons of muscle and are a major endurance-building exercise. That said, there is one thing you should know about lunges: They can be tough on your knees if done incorrectly. If you have bad knees to begin with, skip them and substitute a free squat or leg press if you're at the gym. The key to saving your knees during this exercise is to not let your knee move forward toward your toe line. Keep your knee over your ankle on the leg you are putting most weight on (the front leg) and you should be fine. If you get a dull ache over the front of your knee joint, reassess your technique with the pictures above and make sure your form is correct. To increase the benefit of these lunges, a bicep curl has been added to the mix.

We are using a step-back lunge to further protect your knees. Begin by stepping back with one leg, land on the ball of your back foot with your ankle up and off the ground, and sink down until your front leg thigh is just above parallel to the ground. Then stand up and complete the bicep curl, return to your starting position and repeat on the other leg.

Targets: Glutes, Quads, Biceps, Core
Complete: 2 to 3 Sets of 12 Reps on each leg

Exercise 2
Bridge with Leg Lifts

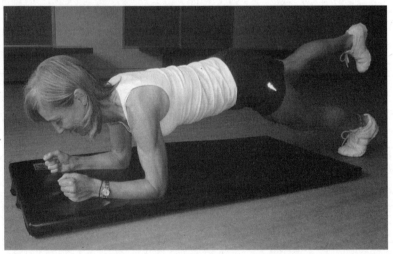

Bridges and planks are excellent overall abdominal and core exercises. They are vital to a proper physical activity program because they help strengthen the musculature that stabilizes the spine during all activity — be it cardio, resistance training, walking around the house, or even sitting at your desk. Keep bridges in your exercise program and you will be able to enjoy a much wider array of exercises for pretty much the rest of your life!

This bridge further tests you with an alternating leg lift to strengthen your core, tighten your tummy, and improve your posture even faster. Begin by supporting yourself on your elbows and toes on a soft surface. Draw your stomach in toward your spine and alternate lifting each leg one to two inches off the ground for one second each. Eventually, you should try to hold the bridge for up to a minute or more, but you can start by just trying to complete five to six lifts per leg per set.

Targets: Abs, Glutes, Chest, Hip Flexors
Complete: 3 Sets of 5 to 6+ Lifts (you can do up to 20 lifts) per leg

Exercise 3
Perform cardio option from list above for 5-10 minutes or more.

Day 4
Exercise 1
Sumo Squats with Lateral Raises

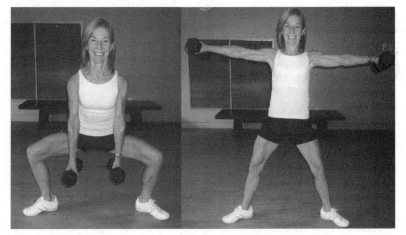

Sumo squats may not sound like the type of exercise you would want to do for your physique, however, the name is completely misleading. This exercise will get your glutes, inner thighs, quads, and hamstrings in great shape all at the same time. This is one of the best lower-body exercises for toning and strengthening the major leg muscles. It is also very mild on your joints. The squats are accompanied by a lateral raise to get a little upper body involvement for added calorie burning and cardiovascular benefit. This is also a great exercise to really work on getting in some big, deep, refreshing breaths.

Start in a wide-leg stance with your toes pointing out on a 45 degree angle with the weights in front of you. Drop down into a "bow legged" squat while keeping your back almost vertical with the weights. Then stand up, squeeze your glutes together and raise your dumbbells out to your sides until your arms are just under parallel to the ground. Keep a slight bend in your elbows at all times. You may need a lighter set of dumbbells for this exercise, so feel free to use 3 to 5 pound dumbbells if necessary to complete the lateral raises with proper form.

Targets: Glutes, Quads, Inner Thighs, Lateral Shoulders
Complete: 3 Sets of 12 to 15 Reps

Exercise 2
Side to Side Crunches with Legs Up

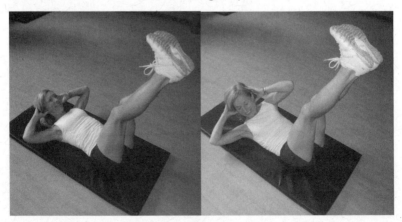

Abdominal muscles (Abs) play a key role in maintaining our ability to balance, breathe, and perform safe, coordinated movements during all our various daily activities. Lean, strong abs are a must for anyone looking to maintain an active, vibrant lifestyle.

This advanced abdominal exercise targets all the major abdominal muscle groups, including rectus femoris (your six-pack), the obliques (love handles), and transverse abdominis (the underlying foundational abdominal muscle that flattens out your lower abs).

Begin by lying on your back with your legs comfortably bent in the air. Draw your stomach in toward your spine and crunch up to one side, return down to the middle, and repeat on the other side. Try to crunch out enough to the side so that you can see down the outside of your leg on each side and maintain a smooth, controlled pace during this exercise — no bobbing and weaving. Finally, breathe out as you crunch up to each side and in on the way down to ensure the deepest possible abdominal contractions during each rep of this exercise.

Targets: Six-Pack and Love Handles (Rectus Abdominus
                 and Internal and External Obliques)
Complete: 3 Sets of 20-25 Reps

Exercise 3
Perform cardio option from list above for 5 to 10 minutes or more.

Day 5
Exercise 1
Lying Inner Thigh Leg Lifts

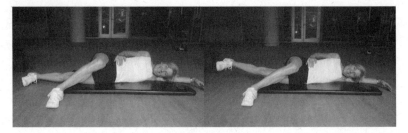

Inner thighs are one of the most important spinal and pelvic stabilizers that help us balance during physical activities and avoid falls. They should be addressed in every exercise program to ensure we are able to stay active and in shape as we age. So, in a roundabout way, having well-toned, strong inner thighs would provide a big part of the background to an active, healthy lifestyle and a fit heart — not to mention very aesthetically pleasing legs.

Begin this exercise by lying on your side with your upper leg crossed in front of your lower knee. Lift your lower leg 1 to 1.5 feet (30-45 cm) off the ground and squeeze your lower inner thigh at the high point of each rep.

Targets: Inner Thighs and Obliques
Complete: 3 Sets of 15 to 20 Reps per leg

Exercise 2
Cobras

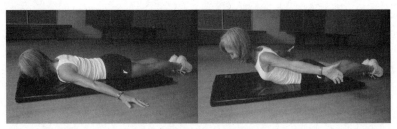

Cobras are a crucial functional exercise for the upper and mid back. This exercise helps keep our ribcage and spinal muscles functioning optimally. It is also "The Hunchback Cure" exercise. Cobras help keep your shoulders back, ribcage in line, and upper spine strong to help you maintain better posture and more efficient and less obstructed breathing — all incredibly good things for your heart. Cobras essentially keep your airways and many of your upper body blood vessels in the best possible positions for optimal flow and function.

Begin on your stomach with your forehead touching the floor and your hands palms down at your sides. Start each rep by slowly lifting your head and upper chest 5 to 6 inches (12-15 cm) off the ground in conjunction with your arms. Keep your arms parallel to the ground while rotating your thumbs laterally until you feel a tight muscle contraction in your mid back and in the back of your upper arms. Keep your head down during every rep and keep your eyes focused on the floor (we do not want you curling your head up and back).

Targets: Postural Back Muscles and Triceps
Complete: 3 Sets of 15 Reps

Exercise 3
Perform cardio option from list above for 5 to 10 minutes or more.

Overexercising — What to Know

There is an expression that starts, "Too much of a good thing ..." Exercise can fall into this category as well. Too much exercise is when we push our joints, systems, and hearts past a healthy endurance. Over-exercising creates free radicals that wreak cellular havoc, and cause decreased immunity; the body uses all its resources up during workouts and has less energy to fight off infectious bugs. Regular exercise, both aerobic and anaerobic (weight bearing), are without a doubt important for heart health. But too much, too fast can put much strain on the heart, resulting in a greater chance of a heart attack. In fact, this is just what was reported in a study presented at the 2003 Physiological Society's conference at the University of Cambridge in the United Kingdom. Sudden bursts of strenuous activity resulted in longer recovery times after the activity, with higher heart rates lasting up to one hour. In contrast, gentler, more moderate exercise allowed the heart rate to return to normal in 15 minutes. This shorter period limits the amount of time in which heart problems can occur. The researchers concluded that exercise training, whereby exercise is regulated, was important for heart disease patients.

Day 6

Exercise 1

Side-to-Side Stationary Lunges

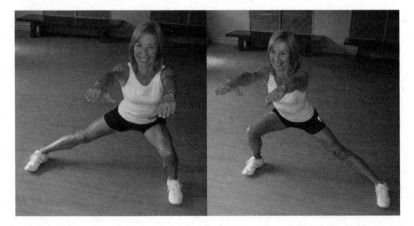

Side lunges combine all the lower body toning and tightening benefits of regular lunges with the added bonus of a little inner thigh attention. This challenging lower body exercise targets all major leg muscles and will help you build lean, toned, and balanced legs. This and all the other leg exercises will also help improve blood flow and supply to your lower body.

Begin in a wide stance with your feet pointing straight ahead and your arms at your sides. Start sinking toward one side while simultaneously reaching forward with your arms and driving your hips backward until your bent upper thigh is just above parallel from the ground. Make sure your bent leg knee stays within the lateral edge line of your shoe when glancing down on it from above and does not "swing outside" your shoe. Press out of the lunge on one side and repeat on the other. You can also drop your hands at the top of each rep and re-extend them as you sink down for a more rhythmic and balanced motion.

Targets: Quads, Glutes, Inner thighs, Hamstrings
Complete: 3 Sets of 10 Reps each leg

Exercise 2
High Hip Lifts off Chair/Bench

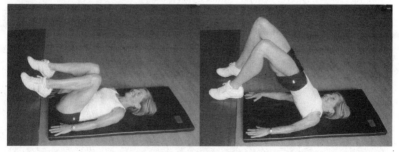

This modified hip lift targets the hamstrings right at the gluteal fold (where the hamstrings meet the butt muscle). Though this exercise is often used for "spot tightening," its true benefits lie in its ability to balance out the tension and contraction strength of the hamstrings in relation to the quadriceps. Having a strength balance between your quads and hamstrings will allow you to perform more activity more efficiently, further enhancing your ability to boost your health and vitality. In short, it means you are going to "lift your butt," balance your lower body to prolong your physical prowess, and burn a ton of calories.

Start by lying on the floor as closely as you can to the apparatus that you are going to use for this exercise. Make sure the object you use is braced against the wall or something that is not going to allow it to move and slide away from you. Place the center of your feet on the edge of the equipment and drive your hips up into the air as high as you can. Once you reach your high point, drop down five to six inches, then drive back up again to complete the rep.

Targets: Glutes and Hamstrings
Complete: 3 Sets of 10 to 12 Reps

Exercise 3
Perform cardio option from list above for 5 to 10 minutes or more.

Day 7
Exercise 1
Front Squat with 1/2 Shoulder Press

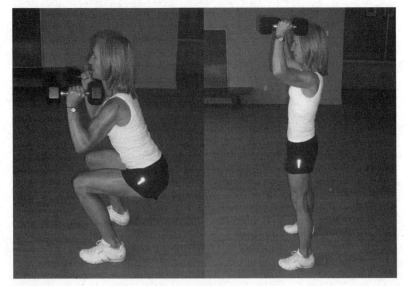

This modified squat will challenge your lower and upper body in a few different movement patterns that you run into and use daily. This exercise is also good for mildly offsetting upper body structural issues such as frozen shoulders and forward head posture, which will help maintain proper neck and upper back circulation and ease of breathing.

Begin with your dumbbells at the top of a bicep curl with the weights in the "hammer swinging hand position." Keep your head up, eyes forward and squat down to just above 90 degrees. Then stand up and press the weights up one to two inches above your head level, then return to the starting position to complete the rep. Make sure to keep a "ski slope" arched back position as you squat down during every rep of this exercise.

Targets: Quads, Glutes, Hamstrings
Complete: 3 Sets of 12 Reps

Exercise 2
Mountain Climbers

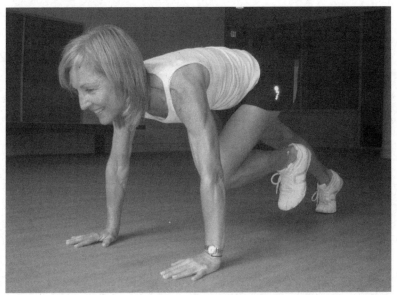

After 30 seconds of this great total body exercise, you will probably feel like you have ascended a small mountain. But if you keep at it, you will be climbing Everest (or a small neighborhood mountain) before you know it! This exercise gives you a great cardio and core workout and it is excellent at building muscular endurance and coordination.

Begin in the same position in which you would perform a push-up and bring one knee forward as if you are in the starting blocks for a running race. Try to keep your back parallel to the ground while you are switching your legs back and forth as fast as you can. In other words, work on avoiding bobbing up and down at the hips each time you switch your leg position.

Targets: Core, Hip Flexors, Quads
Complete: 3 Sets of 25 to 40 Seconds

Exercise 3
Perform cardio option from list above for 5 to 10 minutes or more.

Day 8
Exercise 1
Skull Crushers in Hip Lift Position

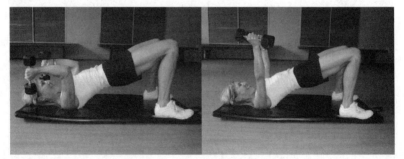

This total body core and balance exercise targets the back of your arms and your glutes while challenging a host of other major muscle groups to play a supportive role. Keep this exercise up on a regular basis and you will tighten two trouble spots on your body and see your lower back function improve as well.

Start on your upper back on the floor, hips and lower back at the top of a hip lift and your dumbbells straight up above you. Make sure you use weights you can fully control as they will be passing by your head during this exercise and you don't want to give yourself a bump on the head.

While maintaining your hips at the top of the hip lift, slowly drop the dumbbells down to the sides of your head while keeping your elbows pointing straight up. As your weights near an inch from the floor, extend them back up until your arms are straight again to complete each rep.

Targets: Triceps, Core, Glutes, Hamstrings
Complete: 3 Sets of 10-12 Reps

Exercise 2
Knee to Opposite Elbow Bridge
on Bench/Couch/Chair/Stairs

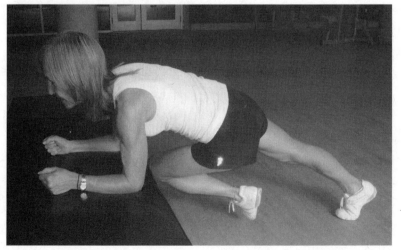

This is another excellent functional exercise for your body that provides various postural improvements and targets many fundamental core muscles. This exercise should be done on a padded surface to comfort your elbows.

Begin by forming a slightly upwardly peaked bridge or plank between your elbows and toes. Draw your stomach in and lift one leg off the ground and bring it diagonally across your body to your opposite elbow and touch, return to starting position and repeat on the other side. Make sure you do not bend at the waist to help your knee touch the opposite elbow — it is best to hold a straight body position and stretch as far as you can without bending. Do not worry if you cannot touch your elbow at first; this will improve over time.

Targets: Core, Chest, Hip Flexors, Arms
Complete: 3 Sets of 8 to 10 Elbow Touches per leg

Exercise 3
Perform cardio option from list above for 5 to 10 minutes or more.

Day 9
Exercise 1
Step-ups with Front Raises

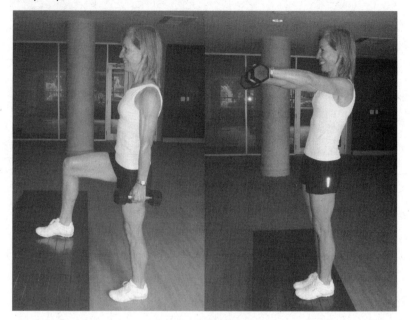

This exercise targets all the major muscles groups to give you a great cardiovascular workout. To ensure your safety during this exercise, use a well-grounded object to step up on, like the bottom stair of a staircase or a proper bench at the gym.

Begin by placing one foot up on the bench. Make sure the leg you have up is at about 90 degrees of flexion at the knee. Step up in a controlled, smooth motion and perform a front raise once you are on the bench. If you're a beginner, it's best to start this exercise on a low bench (approx. 1 foot (30 cm) off the ground or 1 stair at home). Once you complete one step up and front raise on one leg, step down and repeat the same motion on the other side. Alternate on each leg to complete the set and simply carry the dumbbells if your arms tire before your legs do.

Targets: Quads, Glutes, Anterior Shoulders, Hamstrings
Complete: 3 Sets of 8 to 10 each leg

Exercise 2
Moderate Range Windshield Wipers

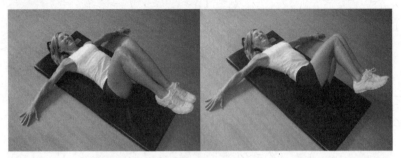

Wipers are a great twisting exercise that challenges your core and keeps your body from losing rotational range. They also tighten and tone the oblique (side stomach) muscles. Adding wipers to your routine should help you maintain a flexible spine with good rotational strength.

Begin on your back on the floor with your knees pointing to the ceiling and lower legs relaxed. With your arms out to each side, slowly tilt your knees laterally to one side until you reach approximately six inches (15 cm) from the floor. Then tilt back to the other side in the same motion your windshield wiper moves. Keep in mind the goal of this exercise is not to eventually touch the floor on each side, it is more to maintain controlled motion and build muscular endurance. As you improve, you can straighten your legs out to add extra challenge to this exercise.

Targets: Obliques and Hip Flexors
Complete: 3 Sets of 10 Reps on each side

Exercise 3
Perform cardio option from list above for 5 to 10 minutes or more.

Day 10
Exercise 1
Bent One-leg Hip Lifts

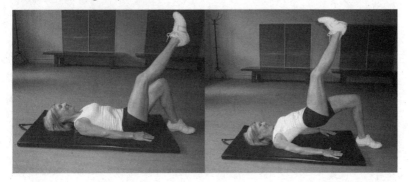

This exercise is a more challenging version of the two-leg hip-lifting motions we discussed earlier. It will take your lower body endurance, circulation, and conditioning to a new level, plus, it will tighten and tone the backs of your thighs. You may only be able to do a few repetitions per leg the first time you try this exercise but, over time, your conditioning will improve rapidly, as will your physique, from this great hamstring and glute lower-body exercise.

Begin on your back on the floor with one leg bent at about 90 degrees with the foot flat on the ground, and the other leg comfortably bent straight up in the air. Drive your hips and lifted leg up into the air as high as you can until your hips form a straight line between your shoulders and knees if looked at from the side. Drop back down and touch the ground for a split second to complete the rep and repeat. Complete all the reps you can on one leg, then switch to the other and repeat.

Targets: Glutes and Hamstrings
Complete: 3 Sets of 8 to 12 Reps on each leg

Exercise 2
Side-to-Side Abdominal Twists

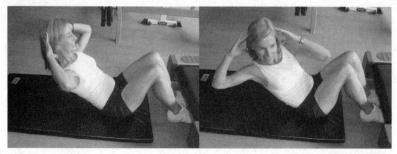

This exercise challenges all your superficial and deep abdominal muscles and forces them to control a great deal of momentum while under load. Beginners can try this exercise without the dumbbell until they are stronger and comfortable with this motion.

Begin by sitting on a soft, padded surface like a pillow on the carpet or a mat at the gym, with your feet hooked under a solid object. Lean back to about 45 degrees and make sure your upper body is in a straight line from your hips to your shoulders. While clasping one dumbbell with both hands, slowly turn from side to side. You only need to rotate about 60 to 80 degrees to each side for optimal benefit. You are not trying to increase range per se in this exercise; you are looking to add more reps and build endurance. As you improve, you can also add more speed for increased challenge.

Targets: Core and Hip Flexors
Complete: 2 Sets of 30 Seconds

Exercise 3
Perform cardio option from list above for 5 to 10 minutes or more.

Conclusion

This is a daily program and will yield best results if performed every day. When you are starting out, feel free to take a break at any time during the program to catch your breath and listen to your body. Go at your own pace and, if you need to skip a day, go ahead and allow your body to recover.

Upon completing the 10-day program, take one day off for recovery, then repeat the program. You can also perform it in reverse to add variety to your day. However, for best results, it is best to avoid other modifications such as mixing and matching exercises.

Your goal with this program should be to reach a point where every single exercise is too easy to challenge you. At this point, feel free to contact me (Byron Collyer) through my Web site for upgrades and additional information on this healthy-heart resistance training program. Best of health!

11. How to Tame Stress

"If wrinkles must be written upon our brows,
let them not be written upon the heart.
The spirit should not grow old."
— James A. Garfield

Let's face it. Stress is inevitable. But what is not inevitable is our response to it, and how this impacts our heart and our overall health.

Imagine the following scenario. You are driving to work and you are rear-ended. You jump out of your car, shaken, annoyed, and when you see your bashed-in bumper, your temper catches hold. What follows is an unhappy confrontation with the apologetic guilty party as you exchange phone numbers, driver's licenses and insurance information. Because you are running late, you finish up quickly, but your bad mood lasts all day.

Here is an alternative scenario involving the same car accident. When you are hit from behind, you do a self-check and realize you are uninjured. Relieved, you get out of your car and ensure that the guilty party is also all right and did not strike you because she was having a health crisis at the wheel. Your bashed-in bumper is upsetting but, you acknowledge, it could have been worse. As you exchange information with the woman, you accept her stricken apology as genuine because you have had a few close calls yourself and you can sympathize with the guilt she is clearly feeling. You finish up and drive to work, grateful that the damage is fixable and that nobody got hurt.

Clearly, these two scenarios represent different ways of thinking about and responding to the same potentially stress-inducing incident. In the former, stress and negativity get the upper hand; in the latter, increased objectivity and positivism improve an unfortunate situation.

In both cases, unseen physiological effects are occurring in the body during these kinds of scenarios — and which approach do you think is healthier for the heart? You guessed it. Number two. Short-term, the second type of reaction reduces the risk of a stress-induced cardiac event (heart attack, arrhythmia). Long-term, we are following a type of behavior that reduces the risk of high blood pressure and heart strain. (If you need a refresher on anger and hostility's detrimental effect on the heart, reread Chapter 4.) So how do we cultivate this way of thinking, feeling, and responding? Before we delve into the hows of stress reduction and the value of relaxing, let's discuss the whys.

Fight or Flight: Our Genetic Legacy

Powerful mechanisms such as the fight-or-flight response have evolved through time to allow the body to shift into "survival" mode so we can either fight back or escape a perceived threat. In times of stress, various hormones within the body are secreted to relay orders. In the musculoskeletal system, muscles tense up. The nervous system reconfigures to best preserve and utilize the body's energy stores. Focus is diverted away from areas that are not immediately essential, such as the digestive system, and is diverted toward the heart and brain where adrenaline and noradrenaline speed our reaction time, heart rate, blood pressure, and blood volume pumped from the heart. The heart starts to pound, breathing quickens and becomes shallow, and we may start to sweat. It is no coincidence that these symptoms match those often found during a heart attack episode. That is why acute stress has short-term and long-term implications for cardiovascular health. Stress can also trigger anxiety attacks, which are sometimes mistaken for heart attacks (see page 65).

As well, other stress hormones relay messages to boost sugar, triglyceride, and cholesterol levels in the blood. The blood gets sticky in case we are injured and need to form clots so we are less likely to bleed to death. The immune system responds, ready to protect us. Over the short-term, this hormonal orchestra is designed to perform effectively. Prolonged stress, however, weakens these mechanisms, reducing immunity, causing systemic wear and tear, and creating a host of physical, behavioral, emotional, and cognitive symptoms. Although we are probably not trying to fight off dangerous predators like our ancestors might have been, these same stress responses can occur while we are stuck in traffic jams and conference calls.

♥ Acute Stress and Cardiovascular Health

The tragedy of 9/11 presented researchers with an opportunity to study the impact of acute stress on the cardiovascular system. Almost 2,700 Americans who had completed a Web-based assessment of acute stress prior to the terrorist attacks were reassessed one, two, and three years later. The physicians found that, even after adjusting for various factors, acute stress responses to 9/11 were associated with a 53 percent increased incidence of cardiovascular ailments, including hypertension and heart problems. These findings were reported in the *Archives of General Psychiatry* in 2008.

We are cramming our days full of activities and events. And regardless of what kind of stress we are under, self-imposed or otherwise — be it physical, mental, emotional, or financial — our body perceives it in the same way. The brain categorizes all stress as deserving a fight-or-flight response and signals hormones to act. Over the course of a normal day, we are activating our stress response repeatedly, and this is where the problems lie.

Why We Need to Relax

We could probably all name a few women (or dozens) who are compulsive overachievers, who never seem to slow down, and who claim they do not know how. We may even admire them, and silently wonder why we cannot seem to get our acts together like they have. Console yourself with this knowledge: Over-activity and the compulsions behind it are not heart-healthy — in fact, they are not healthy, period. Nor are they effective long-term.

Take a Stress Test

The following statements determine your happiness level, how you handle stress, and if you think negatively. Check off the situations that apply to you. Then total the points to determine your stress score, categorized below.

I am worried about paying my bills this month.	1
I look at myself in the mirror and think negative thoughts.	3
I am not content with my body.	3
I almost always fake orgasm.	2
I am lonely.	3
I dislike my job.	3
I like my job but have too much work to do.	3
I like my job, but my boss is too demanding.	1
I am always trying to please everyone.	2
I am exhausted but keep going.	3
Sometimes my stomach feels like it has butterflies.	3
I shop to make myself feel better.	1
I have feelings of guilt or anger.	2
I have feelings of inadequacy (not feeling good enough).	3
I am afraid of failure.	2
I have feelings of anxiety or low moods.	2
I feel trapped or that I can't cope sometimes.	3
I crave sugar.	1
I am a single mother/father.	2
I am a university student.	1
I am in an unhappy marriage.	3
I live with an alcoholic or drug abuser.	2
I work shift work.	1
I work too much and don't have enough play time.	1
I get angry with myself.	2
I hold resentment toward my partner.	3
I cannot discuss my sexual desires with my partner.	2
I don't eat regularly (I wait more than four or five hours between meals).	3
I am sick more than three times a year.	1
I lack sexual desire.	1
I smoke.	3
I drink alcohol more than twice a week.	3

I drink too much caffeine.	2
My family and friends are not supportive of the things I do.	2
I am tired all the time.	3
I have friends who take but never give.	2

How Did You Score?

15 or less	You are handling stress but need to find more balance in your life.
16-29	You know you have to make some changes fast. You are at risk of exhaustion.
30 or more	You are highly stressed. You need to adopt strategies to reduce your risk of stress-related disease immediately.

Initially, stress can enhance performance, but after a certain point, you deteriorate into mental fatigue and feel overwhelmed. Your work and mental, emotional, and physical health suffer. The stress can then lead to chest pain, arrhythmia, high blood pressure, stomach problems, sleep disturbances, depression, anger, burnout, overeating, undereating, drug or alcohol abuse, relationship conflicts, social withdrawal, and much more. Stress permeates all aspects of life and is inescapable. The trick is to find a healthy balance that enhances good productivity yet includes regular relaxation.

By training yourself to relax, you are allowing your body and mind a much-needed break from life's rigors. Physiologically, relaxing slows the breathing and heartbeat, and soothes the nervous system. Oxygen requirements decrease, blood pressure eases, the vessels dilate, and blood flows more easily throughout the body. If stress is the poison, relaxation is the antidote — one we should be embracing whole-heartedly. Relaxing also releases endorphins, which are natural mood lifters that induce a sense of well-being.

Combined with changes in diet, exercise, and nutritional supplementation, stress reduction and management is a protective tool against heart disease and future cardiac events. Ironically, knowing we need to relax and allowing ourselves to relax are two very different things. True relaxation involves a passivity and patience that doesn't come easily to many of us. Have you personally "locked in" stress. Consider your body right now. How are you sitting? Focus on your body and identify the areas where you hold tension. Your neck and back, perhaps, from hunching over a computer all day? Your abdomen? Your jaw? Are you frowning, or smiling? Muscle actually has memory that can trigger mood (frowning vs. smiling) and induce physiological changes, including heart rate and breathing. Hence, de-stressing involves calming the mind and body.

Anti-stress Strategies
Deep Breathing

In ayurvedic medicine, the traditional Indian healing system, breathing represents more than just Westernized ideas of increasing lung capacity and blood oxygen. It involves a transfer of energy, a healing exchange with our environment and the greater universe. What a wonderful and appropriate concept when it comes to the health of the heart, an organ that responds to forgiveness, love, laughter, happiness, and joy.

Do you remember the simple breathing exercise you did in Chapter 4? How did you do? How did you feel afterward (ideally, more relaxed and ready to read on)? It goes without saying that everybody breathes; without air pumping in and out of the lungs to distribute throughout the body, we would be in trouble. Yet most people do not give thought to how they breathe.

Do this quick test now. Sit comfortably on a chair. Place one hand on your chest, the other on your belly. Breathe several times. If your chest-bound hand moves more than your belly hand, you are what is known as a thoracic breather; if your belly-bound hand moves more than your chest-bound hand, you are a belly breather. Belly - or diaphragmatic - breathing is what we instinctively did as babies. Besides providing more oxygen to the system, it also allows us to expel more carbon dioxide wastes. Most of us expand our chests when we breathe, which elevates our shoulders and is, in fact, a relatively shallow way of inhaling. Better breathing — belly breathing — pushes the abdomen in and out more forcefully, pumping more oxygen into our system.

Tuning in to how we breathe requires mindfulness and practice — mindfulness in recognizing our breathing patterns and how they change (e.g., during times of stress), and the practice to correct any unhealthy ones. One advantage to deep breathing is that you can ease into it any time, any place, anywhere — and the only person who has to know is you. Whether it is during a meeting or in a disagreement with a loved one, there is no wrong time to take a moment, reflect, then purposefully adjust. This breathing mechanism also encourages us to tune in to our bodies in general. Human beings, and women in particular, often miss those subtle messages that are being sent from within.

Mindful breathing is a habit to cultivate as much as possible. Do it daily, at whatever time and in whatever form suits you. The general rule is, breathe in and out through your nose (not your mouth). Breathe deeply and regularly, eyes closed, with intention and inward focus. Some people find that it helps to envision the breathing as waves, encroaching and receding.

Breathing exercise 1
Close your eyes. Whisper "ha" and feel the sound as it resonates in the back of your throat.

Close your mouth and breathe in through your nose, regularly and smoothly. As you breathe in, feel the air striking the back roof of your mouth.

Exhale while silently vocalizing the "ha" sound, experiencing it resonate in your throat. Your breath should be light, unforced, like gentle snoring.

Place your hand on your belly to ensure belly breathing (versus chest breathing). On the exhale, contract your belly muscles to ensure all air is expelled.

Repeat for two or three minutes.

♥ Set the Relaxation Stage

Create your special place. It could be an unused room in your house, a sunny spot in the front yard, or a cushioned corner of your bedroom. Anywhere away from the phone or TV will do. Designate this area for relaxation and use it routinely.

Comfort first. Who can relax if they are taut with tension and holding themselves upright? Choose a comfortable chair, a pillowed seat on the floor, or whatever works for you. Your clothing should be equally unconstrained. Note: If you are on the verge of falling asleep, you are too comfortable!

Time it out. Insomniacs are often encouraged to create bedtime routines. Likewise for relaxation. Choose a time of day that works for you and create a relaxation routine. Do your best to stay regular, but if you cannot, do not inwardly beat yourself up about it.

Practice, practice, practice. Routine relaxation, once per day or more, will induce the best overall effect. You will become attuned to your body, mind and emotions, while simultaneously lowering your blood pressure and heart rate, and protecting against stress effects.

Forgive your wandering mind. Learning to relax is like any other skill. It takes practice. As you try to focus inwardly, you will find your mind drifting to random thoughts. Your internal self is a chatterbox. Rather than fight these spurts, allow them to form, then let them go and refocus. Accept your own role in the process. Do not judge yourself, and you will find that relaxation comes to you.

Breathing exercise 2
This one is great at work. Sit at your desk, your back straight, feet flat on the floor.

Eyes closed, inhale slowly and deeply, focusing on the expansion of your belly (leave your hand on your belly if necessary). As you exhale slowly through your nose, make a low humming sound in your throat.

Repeat for two to three minutes.

Breathing exercise 3
The key to this one is in the exhalation. Exhale and inhale fully as per breathing exercise 1. Then, using your abdominal muscles, exhale spurts of air at a rate of about two per second. Exhale forcefully but with control about fifteen times. If you experience discomfort, reduce the exhalations or resume your normal breathing.

Repeat three cycles interspersed with cycles of breathing exercise 1. Always finish with a full, gentle exhale, inhale, exhale.

If ever you feel dizzy, return to your normal breathing until you feel better. Always finish with a few moments of relaxing to transition back into the real world. Some people may experience a slight lightheadedness, so wait peacefully until it passes.

Yoga: Ancient Practice Has Heart
More than 5,000 years old, yoga unites body, mind, and spirit, and also combines elements of relaxation, guided imagery, visualization, and meditation. Yoga comes in several forms. "Hatha yoga," which focuses on gentle stretching poses and supportive breathing, is best suited to relaxation purposes and breaking down the muscle patterns of stress. Hatha yoga will not result in the same ultra-sweaty state as power "ashtanga" or hot-room "bikram" yoga, but that is okay. Relaxation is your purpose here.

Regular yoga improves mood, circulation, digestion, breathing, immunity, flexibility, and muscle tone. A recent study including yoga practice for cancer patients confirmed several heart-supportive effects as well. Fifty-nine cancer patients followed an eight-week "mindfulness-based stress reduction" program, including relaxation, meditation, and gentle yoga that was found to reduce stress symptoms, inflammatory markers, cortisol levels, and systolic blood pressure. Conversely, immunity and mood improved.

Another study focused on 10 patients with cardiovascular disease and 23 without that were part of a six-week program involving 90-minute yoga and meditation sessions, three times a week. These sessions were shown to improve the function of the endothelial cells lining arteries by 69 percent. Regardless of whether the participants had heart disease or not, their blood pressure, resting heart rate, and body mass index decreased during the study period. Long-term yoga practice (for one year or more) is also associated with increased insulin sensitivity, and has been found beneficial for patients with chronic heart failure, by lowering inflammation markers and improving quality of life.

Considering Surgery? Consider Integrative Medicine.

A recent study on heart disease management gives a new meaning to "prepping for surgery." Sixteen cardiac patients took antioxidants coenzyme Q10 and alpha-lipoic acid, magnesium, and omega-3 essential fatty acids for 36 days prior to their operations. They also followed mild exercise and stretching regimens, and practiced music, stress reduction, and relaxation therapies. Prior to surgery, they reported improvements in physical health, mental health, and quality of life scores. Four weeks after surgery, these benefits continued. In contrast, another group who did not practice integrative medicine experienced declines in all three areas. "A program of combined metabolic, physical and mental preparation before cardiac surgery," the authors of *Heart, Lung and Circulation* wrote, "is safe, feasible and may improve quality of life, lower systolic blood pressure, reduce levels of oxidative stress and thus has the potential to enhance post-operative recovery."

Meditate Stress Away

You do not have to sit on a rock, or be cross-legged and bald, to meditate. The practice of meditation has evolved past old stereotypes into a modality with applications well-suited to modern life. You may recall that depression is one of several psychosocial factors that increases the risk of heart disease. In 2009, the first large clinical trial investigated the effect of psychosocial intervention on the heart. Two hundred and eight patients with heart failure were followed for a year after eight weeks of training in meditation, coping skills, and support group discussion. Compared to a control group, the participants reported lower anxiety and depression, and improved symptoms of heart failure, even at the one-year mark.

The combination of meditation and breathing generated positive effects in a recent randomized pilot trial involving 52 patients who did not receive pharmaceutical treatment for high blood pressure. Those who underwent eight weeks of meditation and breathing techniques "induced clinically relevant and consistent decreases in heart rate, systolic and diastolic blood pressure." A 2006 study noted that yoga with meditation improved endothelial function in people with coronary artery disease, and that this combination resulted in significant reductions in blood pressure, heart rate, and body mass index in the 33 subjects, whether they had existing heart disease or not. In a randomized, controlled trial of 103 heart disease patients, transcendental meditation for 16 weeks improved blood pressure, insulin resistance, and cardiac autonomic nervous system tone compared to a control group receiving health education.

Suggested Meditation Resources

Practical Meditation for Busy Souls (2007) by Margo Adair & William Aal, book + CD

Still the Mind: Simple Breathing Practices for Inner Peace (2008) by Bodhipaksa, 2 CDs

The Beginner's Guide to Meditation (2006) by Joan Borysenko, 2 CDs

Meditations for Relaxation and Stress Reduction (2005) by Joan Borysenko, 1 CD

Daily Meditations for Calming Your Anxious Mind (2008) by Jeffrey Brantley & Wendy Millstine, paperback

Mindfulness for Beginners (2006) by Jon Kabat-Zinn, audio book (CD)

Wherever You Go There You Are: Mindfulness Meditation in Everyday Life (2004) by Jon Kabat-Zinn, audio book (CD)

Meditation for Dummies (2006) by Stephan Bodian, paperback

Simple Meditation Exercise

Sit somewhere quiet and peaceful where you will not be disturbed and are less likely to be distracted. Use a chair or flat pillow.

Calm your mind with a few diaphragmatic breaths. Focus on your breathing, the in and out movement of your belly.

If you prefer, mentally focus on a neutral word or phrase, e.g., Love, Live, Peace, Joy, Relax. Words to avoid include those that sound like commands, e.g., Go, Stop, Wait.

Your mind may wander, especially as you are learning your technique. Allow it to happen, then return your attention to your breathing or word.

During this time, not just thoughts but judgements, sensations, images, memories, and desires might arise. Acknowledge them, accept them as part of the process, then refocus on your breathing. Without force, these random distractions will disappear by themselves.

Set an alarm clock nearby to keep you on track. Start with 5 minutes. Gradually continue your meditation time until you are at 20 minutes.

Finish with a few belly breaths.

Above all, avoid preconceptions of what meditation should be. Be positive about the process. There is one very good reason why mind-body therapies, including guided imagery, meditation, progressive muscle relaxation (see Chapter 12), yoga, tai chi, and qigong are used by 17 percent of people with medical problems. Because they work.

12. Think Happy, Live with Heart

*"One of the hardest things in life is having words
in your heart that you can't utter."*
— James Earl Jones

Try this experiment. Spend a few uninterrupted moments thinking about your last tropical vacation. Maybe you spent your days lazing on a towel in the sand, feeling the heat beat down, the lulling sound of waves nearby, the mood dozy, peaceful, content. All your daily troubles were far away; the only thing crossing your mind on occasion was what to eat for dinner ... Even though you might not realize it, your body is right now responding to this image. Do you feel a little more relaxed, your neck muscles looser? Has a smile inadvertently formed on your face?

The things we imagine, dream about, or remember (whether it is positive or negative) actually impact our physical self on a cellular level. Many professional athletes and Olympic contenders use this technique — they envision success to help them achieve their goals. Sports psychology is a huge industry; a good sports psychologist who can guide a team to a championship is worth her weight in gold. Athletes like golfer Tiger Woods are famed for their mental drive. But even if we are not athletes, we can harness this mind-body connection to help us let go of stress and heal our bodies.

In the last chapter, we talked about the importance of stress reduction, in conjunction with the Heart Health Diet, exercise, and targeted nutritional supplementation. Deep breathing, yoga, and meditation are just three techniques that soothe the physiological mechanisms that accompany stress and contribute to elevated blood pressure, cortisol, and other markers that set the stage for cardiovascular wear and tear, cholesterol deposition, and heart disease. Visualization (imagery) is another powerful tool that each of us can access within ourselves. In a way, cause and effect starts in our brain. And guiding our thoughts is an important step in life, and in health.

Visualization has proven helpful in reducing pre-surgery anxiety and post-operative pain, in managing other types of pain, in reducing stress and cortisol levels, and in reducing cravings — to mention just a few of the most recent studies. Its effect on immunity is remarkable. In a recent randomized, controlled trial, for instance, 80 women with breast cancer underwent chemotherapy followed by surgery, radiotherapy, and hormone therapy. Those in a mind-body intervention group were taught relaxation and guided imagery. They also kept diaries on the frequency of relaxation practice and imagery vividness. Immunological cell activity was checked 10 times over 37 weeks. Researchers found that those women who had engaged in relaxation and guided imagery had significantly higher activity levels of several key immune responses. In other words, guided imagery and relaxation enhanced the women's anti-cancer defenses. A recent study also confirmed the benefits of using post-stroke visualization for quicker recuperation. Stroke patients who used mental imagery had significantly enhanced relearning of daily tasks and performance compared to a group who received only conventional functional rehabilitation.

Visualisation (guided imagery) can be practiced alone, accompanied by a CD or tape, or with a health professional. Everyone and anyone can benefit from it. There is no right or wrong way to visualize, although the more senses we use, the better it seems to work. It may also help if you personalize the image you use. If you like gardening, for example, create a visualization about being in your special outdoor place, one with nature.

♥ Guided Imagery:
- Reduces stress and anxiety
- Improves sleep
- Speeds recovery
- Decreases blood pressure
- Decreases pain

Healing Heart Visualization

This visualization would work for any body part, but keep in mind that it is a sample exercise. There are many excellent visualization techniques available in books on this subject.

On a piece of paper, create a graphic of the body part in question. Since you are reading this book, the problem likely lies somewhere in your cardiovascular system. If you have a blocked artery, where does the blockage occur? Shade or circle the area on the paper. If your heart is weak in a specific area, do the same. Keep in mind that this is your visualization, yours, and yours alone. If it is meaningful for you to visualize your heart as the red image we all grew up drawing for Valentine's Day, that is fine. Or you might be drawn to an encyclopedic depiction of the heart in all its complicated glory, or you might ask your cardiologist for specific details to incorporate into your image. It is less important to have a perfect, anatomically correct visual than it is to create one that resonates with you personally.

Now that you have your "before" image prepared, mentally create an "after" image. If you have arrhythmia, envision a steadily beating heart. If your blood pressure is too low, perhaps your image is a pulsing heart that can push blood through the system without problem. Clogged arteries? Imagine smooth arteries unlined with plaque. You get the idea. And if you do not have a specific heart problem, just visualize your version of a healthy heart. If you also want to draw the "after" image on a separate sheet of paper for reference, go right ahead.

Warm up with the meditation exercise on page 230, then ease into your healing-heart visualization. Envision your "before" picture transforming into your "after" picture. A popular technique is using white light. With each breath, envision yourself deeply inhaling pure, bright light. This light is healing, soothing, and pushes out all stress and "before" images as it fills you. Gradually, envision the healing light easing down your chest and congregating around your heart (or around any other injured/troubled area). As you exhale, imagine black light (negative energy) associated with that area being emitted out of your pores, or the soles of your feet, or other exit points. Let go of all concerns, worries, tension, anxiety, and fear in the black light or smoke that leaves your body and dissipates into the universe. Repeat until all blackness is gone and your "after" picture is fully in place, surrounded by clean, white energy.

A healing visualization exercise can be as short as a minute or two. Always finish a visualization with several deep, diaphragmatic breaths. Slowly open your eyes and get up when you are ready. Some people also enjoy simple stretching to reaccustom the body to activity.

Do You Live with Heart?

If you are familiar with Dr. Dean Ornish's work with heart disease, you may recall his discussions about how some people with heart disease, when asked to visualize their hearts, report that there is a wall or fortress around them. Interestingly, Dr. Ornish contends that this represents a disassociation between people's feelings and experiences, or between thoughts and feelings. Intuitively, is there not something very real about this idea? For sure, many of us have a hard time acknowledging our feelings to ourselves, let alone expressing them to others. And yet living with heart requires exactly that.

The heart is more than just an organ with a job to do. Sometimes, in the rush of modern life, as we are racing to work, to meet friends, to catch a plane, to meet a deadline, to make it to the video store before closing, we forget to appreciate this fact. Each of us, even the most enlightened, has to be occasionally reminded about the need to nurture ourselves from the outside in. Unhealthy thoughts and emotions like grief, hurt, and anger can take an unhappy toll on the cardiovascular system and overall health. Conversely, "living with heart" not only cultivates happiness, balance, passion and a more positive outlook, it also sends powerful messages at a cellular level that impact your physical health.

Have a Positive Outlook

We are what we think. Our thoughts, judgments, wishes, dreams, and experiences color our vision of the world. They can put an overcast day on the verge of sunlight, or on the verge of a thunderstorm. From the moment we wake until the moment we fall asleep, thousands of thoughts fill our minds, and influence our actions and our moods. These are all intricately connected and, in turn, affect our health. So how do we break patterns of negativity and set ourselves on the positive path? For starters, we can retrain our thoughts, just like we can reprogram our patterns of eating, exercising, sitting, sleeping, breathing, and driving.

Identify negative thoughts.

These are often split-second mental reactions to an incident/scenario. They may involve "red flag" words like *should, never, must, always.*

Stop and breathe.

Visualize the word "stop" or say "stop" aloud. Allow yourself several moments to mentally step back and take a few deep belly breaths.

Reflect and redirect.

When you are calmer, it is easier to be objective. Consider the situation again, and ask yourself, what is fact, what is subjectivity? Then modify your thoughts. If your initial thought, for instance, was an anxious, *I'll never finish this project,* your new thought might be, *I can do it, one step at a time.*

Keep practicing.

Retraining the brain will take time. It is a skill, just like dancing. Forgive yourself any setbacks, and congratulate yourself on your successes.

Positive to bed, positive to rise.

Before bed and after arising, say a quick affirmation, or more than one. Spoken words are very powerful; the subconscious mind accepts them and

♥ Affirmations with Heart

If there is one standout woman who's done more for our awareness of the power of thoughts and their role in self-healing and success, it is Louise Hay. Since the early 1980s, this bestselling author has been an inspiration. She teaches that we are all responsible for all our experiences, and that every thought we think creates our future. At all times, we have power within us. Through resentment, criticism, guilt, and more negativity, we create illness. By loving and accepting ourselves and by forgiving others here and now, we create positive changes that dissolve disease and heal our lives.

Below are a select few affirmations for heart-related conditions that she lists in her book, *You Can Heal Your Life*, which is a must on every bookshelf. Write them on a Post-it note and stick them on your bathroom mirror, fridge door, or computer screen. Repeat them often and include them in your daily morning and bedtime routine, if desired.

Anxiety: "I love and approve of myself and I trust the process of life. I am safe."

Arteriosclerosis: "I am completely open to life and to joy. I choose to see with love."

Blood pressure, high (hypertension): "I joyously release the past. I am at peace."

Blood clotting: "I awaken new life within me. I flow."

Cholesterol, high (atherosclerosis): "I choose to live life. My channels of joy are wide open. It is safe to receive."

Heart problems, general: "My heart beats to the rhythm of love."

Heart attack: "I bring joy back to the center of my heart. I express love to all."

Inflammation: "My thinking is peaceful, calm, and centered."

our bodies respond to them. Affirmations should be strong and powerful. Here are a few examples, although feel free to make up your own:

"I am a cheerful, positive person who embraces life."
"I love my life and embrace each day with happiness."
"My life is full of joy, happiness, and peace."

Surround yourself with support. Share your goal of being positive with family and friends. Ask them to point out when you utter a negative thought.

Fill your life with positive books, DVDs, and music that you can turn to when you need reminding about the power of positive thinking. There is no shortage of well-researched material on this subject.

Laughter: The Best Medicine?

Have you ever gone to a movie and come out with your stomach aching from having laughed so hard? What an amazing feeling. You were also probably happy, talkative, and bubbling with energy. It likely was not a conscious choice to be in a good mood; you simply could not help yourself. Why do you think television's *America's Funniest Home Videos* with Bob Sagat lasted seven seasons, is still in reruns? This humorous classic and others like it never fail to elicit smiles. Such is the power of laughter. It lifts us, inspires us, tranforms us. And when it comes to health, yes, it sounds like a cliché, but it's true: Laughter is truly one of nature's best medicines.

Laughter and smiling reduce the symptoms of depression, physical and emotional pain, and create relationships. When we laugh, the body releases endorphins. These "feel-good" hormones are natural painkillers and bring about the slightly euphoric high that also accompanies a good workout. Laughter relieves stress hormones, improves immunity, and lowers inflammation in the body. According to Japanese studies, laughter even affects blood sugar levels with diabetics who watched a comedy versus a boring lecture experiencing lower spikes in blood sugar.

Laughter also lowers blood pressure via a vasodilator effect confirmed in a 2005 University of Maryland study. The researchers looked at 20 volunteers whose average age was 33, and had normal blood pressure, cholesterol, and blood glucose levels. Each participant watched 15 minutes of two movies intended to evoke extreme emotional responses, such as the opening scene of *Saving Private Ryan* or a segment of a comedy like *King Pin*. They were also shown a movie intended to produce the opposite emotion. Laughter, the researchers found, caused the endothelial cells that line blood vessels to dilate and increase blood flow. Conversely, the stressful film clips caused these cells to constrict and impede blood circulation. Overall, average blood flow increased 22 percent during laughter, and decreased 35 percent during mental stress.

According to Dr. Michael Miller, director of preventive cardiology at the University of Maryland Medical Center and associate professor of medicine at the University of Maryland School of Medicine: "The endothelium is the first line in the development of atherosclerosis or hardening of the arteries, so, given the results of our study, it is conceivable that laughing may be important to maintain a healthy endothelium, and reduce the risk of cardiovascular disease. At the very least, laughter offsets the impact of mental stress, which is harmful to the endothelium." Research has found that the endothelial cells in the arteries have receptors that attract the endorphins generated by laughter. This joining leads to the direct release of nitrous oxide, which relaxes muscles and results in vessel dilation.

Subscribe to laugh a day.
Sign up for a free service like www.ajokeaday.com or www.ahajokes.com, which send free jokes to your email.

Hit the DVD rental store.
Stock up on comedies, sitcoms, and Disney and Pixar classics. (They are not just for kids.)

Humor-ize your screensaver.
Search Google images for funny images, raid your photo albums, or hit your favorite cartoon Web site.

Post laugh reminders.
Make a point of reading the comics in your local paper. Clip out any good ones and post them on your fridge and on your bathroom mirror.

Join a laughter club or laughter yoga.
Yes, there is actually a non-profit group that facilitates the latter: www. laughteryoga.org claims an exercise routine that is "one of the fastest ways to accelerate heart rate and provides an excellent cardiovascular workout and heart massage."

Listen to laughter.
Download audio comedy programs and listen in the car while driving (pull over if you get distracted!) and while traveling. Laughter tracks stimulate our own laughter; it is contagious. Try a background laughter CD or tape at your next party or while doing household tasks.

Self-honesty: Emotions and Expression

In earlier sections, you saw how negative emotions are linked to heart disease. Anger, hostility, anxiety, and depression can worsen cardiovascular troubles. Likewise, when a diagnosis of heart disease is given, it is common to feel shocked, upset, or depressed. However, strong support from those around you and a multidimensional plan like the one in this book can help move you into the next stage: acceptance. Here is where another component of true heart healing — emotional and psychological — lies. Acceptance sets the stage for emotional honesty, which helps us regain/find our sense of self and our purpose in life.

Think of your beating heart right now. What do you envision? Can you see it clearly, pink and vibrant with health and open to all possibilities? Or is the mental picture of your heart hazy, blocked, or

Daily Acts of Kindness

Every day, Ted Kuntz puts three coins in his pocket that he will never spend. In the morning, he slips them into his left pocket, and one by one, as he does something good for another person, he transfers them into his right. "The goal is to have all three coins in the right pocket by the end of the day," says Kuntz.

They're called Kindness Coins, and this motivational speaker, author, psychotherapist, and counselor minted them as a reminder to boost daily acts of kindness.

The concept is probably a familiar one. Actors Kevin Spacey and Haley Joel Osment took it to the big screen in *Pay it Forward*, and Oprah's "gratitude list" urges millions of viewers to shift attention toward the positive of life, and away from the negative.

"Most of us aspire to be peaceful, joyful people, but I don't think we know how to do that. We're taught to be angry and afraid," Kuntz says. "The average person thinks nine times as many negative thoughts as positive ones."

"We're ill-prepared to change and we're waiting for something outside of ourselves when what's really under our power of control is what's in ourselves," he adds.

Kuntz personally knows what it is like to be negative. After his infant son was permanently injured many years ago, he lived in a place of anger, fear, and resentment.

"It was too hard," he recalls of those trying years. "So I began a personal journey to understand how to have more peace and joy in my life."

His book, *Peace Begins with Me*, which received honorable mention by the Independent Book Publishers Association in 2006, has been part of this process and includes insights about how to take responsibility for one's happiness.

The first step, Kuntz says, is acknowledging one's thoughts, noticing how one thinks. After that, he teaches how to use the mind and imagination creatively, rather than reactively, by being able to specifically answer such questions as, "What do I intend?" and "What am I focused on?"

Kuntz suggests that paying attention to one's thoughts is about more than joy and peace; it is also about health.

"Research says the body doesn't distinguish between real and imagined thoughts. Your body comes under the same stress and turmoil as your brain."

Stress, as we have noted, is certainly a serious issue, affecting more than 40 percent of adults. A common statistic indicates that stress-related ailments and complaints account for up to 90 percent of all doctor visits.

Stress, Kuntz tells us, is a fact of life, but we can choose to respond to stress in a positive way, thus reducing the effects of stress and living happier and healthier lives. And in case he forgets, he has those Kindness Coins in his pocket to remind him.

barricaded? The goal is to not only be able to visualize a healthy heart (e.g., by following the techniques on page 235), but also to remove any emotional blockages that prohibit healing and, ultimately, happiness, peace, and joy. We must learn to listen and accept any inner messages, be they good or bad. Are we being emotionally honest with ourselves? Pretend your heart is your best friend; what would your best friend want to say to you? Of course, this level of self-reflection is not always easy. The issues that come to light might be small, for example, forgiving a grievance against an ex-coworker, or large, like dealing with issues of abuse or family trauma. Some people will be able to do this alone, some will need guidance. Whichever way works best for you is acceptable. The only unhealthy technique is continual avoidance.

As you become more emotionally and mentally conscious, you will grow happier, less stressed, and less prone to anxiety and depression.

You are more engaged in life. Naturally, communication is a key factor in this transformation. You must learn to be honest, not only with yourself but also with the people in your life — your partner, siblings, friends, colleagues, and acquaintances. How you express your thoughts and feelings is no simple matter. If you are angry or resentful, you could express it by lashing out verbally, or smothering it inwardly. Maybe you bottle it all in until, one day, you will snap and a bigger explosion occurs. Or maybe you do not do anything and lead a tragic lifetime of negative emotion. Underlying all these "maybes" is the fact that the emotions are the same, but the pattern of behavior is not.

Now that you are determined to live with heart and increase your inward focus, you might also need to make external changes in the way you interact with others. By expressing yourself and listening effectively, you help manage stress, deepen relationships in a meaningful way, and strengthen your sense of self-worth and personal boundaries.

Final Cardio Sense
Phone a friend.
Regular interaction with people who care is essential to a well-balanced life. Loneliness is a major predictor of disease.

Build your support team.
This means some combination of a spouse, family and friends but can also include a support group, religious group, hobby group, and/or various health-care professionals.

Share how you feel and think.
If you have recently been diagnosed with heart disease or its risk factors, the people in your life are going through it as well. Talk with them, share your resources. They may want to help but do not know how. Ask them for what you need support-wise, but it is okay to draw boundaries if you need personal time or if they're overzealous in expressing their opinions of what you should do. Remember, it is your health journey.

Find joy in play. Rediscover your inner child. Lightheartedness enhances immunity, and increases creativity and cheer in all aspects of our lives.

Be grateful.
Before bed each night, express what you are grateful for in your life. People who perform a daily gratitude exercise are more alert, enthusiastic, determined, and optimistic. Grateful people also report having fewer physical complaints and more energy.

Give of yourself.
By focusing outward, you attract abundance. Directing attention away from yourself benefits others and allows you to take a realistic look at how lucky you are. Altruism and compassion deactivate negative emotions that affect your immune, hormone, and cardiovascular systems.

Start a journal.
Writing is a great form of self-expression. Better to write out what you are feeling than to repress it or express it unhealthfully. Writing helps recovery after trauma/emotional upset and also improves health by bolstering certain immune factors.

Listen to music.
Music therapy is a wonderful wellness tool. Play a CD or listen to the radio while you get ready for work, commute, cook, eat, clean, or before bed. Experiment with song writing, performing, developing lyrics. Join a music appreciation club and attend live productions.

Get a pet.
Animals help us relax, lower blood pressure, enhance emotions, and help us deal with change and loss.

Take a nap.
This simple pleasure can improve cardiac health. A daily half-hour mid-day nap cuts heart attack risk by 30 percent. A one-hour nap, by 50 percent.

Have sex.

The intimacy that sensuality and sexuality generate profoundly influence well-being. If you have had a heart attack, check with your doctor about when to resume sexual activity. It is usually within a few weeks. The physical exertion of normal sexual activity is within the range of routine daily activities like brisk walking, golf, or carrying a full bag of groceries. Still, a reintroduction to sex should not be rushed. Interestingly, regular exercise after a heart attack practically eliminates the risk of a reoccurrence during sex. The more you exercise (including having sex), the lower your risk.

A Heart Health Conclusion

If there is one thing that this book hopefully has taught you, it is that you have the power to heal your heart. Armed with knowledge, fueled with determination, you have the power to avoid and reverse heart disease, to get healthy, to make memories count. Live Heart Health and thrive. A healthy diet feeds the body. Supplements improve it. Exercise trains it. Stress reduction calms it. What is left for us is thinking happy and living with heart, an excellent finale by any standards. Lao Tzu, the famous Chinese philosopher and founder of Taoism, once said, "Love is of all passions the strongest, for it attacks simultaneously the head, the heart and the senses." This is our greatest wish for you and your loved ones. Learn to love. Be happy. Live with passion.

References and Resources

Introduction

Harman, N.L. *et al.* "Increased dietary cholesterol does not increase plasma low density lipoprotein when accompanied by an energy-restricted diet and weight loss." *Eur J Nutr.* 2008 Oct; 47(7):408.

"Heart Disease and Stroke Statistics – 2009 Update." Dallas, Texas: American Heart Association; 2009.

Herron, K. *et al.* "High intake of cholesterol results in less atherogenic low-density lipoprotein particles in men and women independent of response classification*1." *Metabolism.* 2004; 53(6): 823-830.

Iglay, H.B. *et al.* "Moderately increased protein intake predominately from egg sources does not influence whole body, regional, or muscle composition responses to resistance training in older people." *J Nutr Health Aging.* 2009; 13(2):108-14.

Heart Disease Risks

American Overweight and Obesity Statistics, Centers for Disease Control and Prevention, Atlanta, GA (www.cdc.gov/obesity/data/index.html).

Angerer, P. *et al.* "Effect of oral postmenopausal hormone replacement on progression of atherosclerosis: a randomized, controlled trial." *Arterioscler Thromb Vasc Biol.* 2001; 21:262–268.

Bairey Merz, C.N. *et al.* "Hypoestrogenemia of hypothalamic origin and coronary artery disease in premenopausal women: a report from the NHLBI-sponsored WISE study." *J Am Coll Cardiol.* 2003; 41:b413–419.

Barrett-Connor, E. "Postmenopausal estrogen and prevention bias." *Ann Intern Med.* 1991; 115: 455–456.

Barrett-Connor, E. "Sex differences in coronary heart disease. Why are women so superior? The 1995 Ancel Keys Lecture." *Circulation.* 1997; 95:252–264.

Barrett-Connor, E., and T.L. Bush. "Estrogen and coronary heart disease in women." *JAMA.* 1991; 265:1861–1867.

Barrett-Connor, E., and D. Goodman-Gruen. "Prospective study of endogenous sex hormones and fatal cardiovascular disease in postmenopausal women." *BMJ.* 1995; 311:1193–1196.

Barrett-Connor, E., and D. Grady. "Hormone replacement therapy, heart disease, and other considerations." *Annu Rev Public Health.* 1998; 19:55–72.

Barrett-Connor, E. *et al.* "Raloxifene and cardiovascular events in osteoporotic postmenopausal women: four-year results from the MORE (Multiple Outcomes of Raloxifene Evaluation) randomized trial." *JAMA.* 2002; 287:847–857.

Barrett-Connor, E. *et al.* "The Postmenopausal Estrogen/Progestin Interventions Study: primary outcomes in adherent women." *Maturitas.* 1997; 27:261–274.

Bibbins-Domingo *et al.* "Adolescent Overweight and Future Adult Coronary Heart Disease." *NEJM.* 2007; 357(23):2371-2379.

Brett, K.M., and J.H. Madans. 1997 Use of postmenopausal hormone replacement therapy: estimates from a nationally representative cohort study. *Am J Epidemiol.*145:536–545.

Burger, H.G. *et al.* "Serum inhibins A and B fall differentially as FSH rises in perimenopausal women." *Clin Endocrinol (Oxf).* 1998; 48:809–813.

Bush, T.L. *et al.* "Cardiovascular mortality and noncontraceptive use of estrogen in women: results from the Lipid Research Clinics Program Follow-up Study." *Circulation.* 1987; 75:1102–1109.

Bush, T.L. *et al.* "Estrogen use and all-cause mortality. Preliminary results from the Lipid Research Clinics Program Follow-Up Study." *JAMA.* 1983; 249:903–906.

Byington, R.P. *et al.* "Effect of estrogen plus progestin on progression of carotid atherosclerosis in postmenopausal women with heart disease: HERS B-mode substudy." *Arterioscler Thromb Vasc Biol.* 2002; 22:1692–1697.

Canadian Overweight and Obesity Statistics, Statistics Canada, http://www.statcan.gc.ca/pub/82-620-m/2005001/article/adultsadultes/8060-eng.htm#1.

Cauley, J.A. *et al.* "Reliability and interrelations among serum sex hormones in postmenopausal women." *Am J Epidemiol.* 1991; 133:50–57.

Cauley, J.A. *et al.* "The relation of endogenous sex steroid hormone concentrations to serum lipid and lipoprotein levels in postmenopausal women." *Am J Epidemiol.* 1990; 132:884–894.

Cherry, N. *et al.* "Oestrogen therapy for prevention of reinfarction in postmenopausal women: a randomized placebo controlled trial." *Lancet.* 2002; 360:2001–2008.

Clarke, S.C. *et al.* "A study of hormone replacement therapy in postmenopausal women with ischaemic heart disease: the Papworth HRT atherosclerosis study." *BJOG.* 2002; 109:1056–1062.

Critchley, J.A., and S. Capewell. "Smoking cessation for the secondary prevention of coronary heart disease." *Cochrane Database of Systematic Reviews.* 2003; Issue 4. Art. No.: CD003041. DOI: 10.1002/14651858.CD003041.pub2.

"Effects of estrogen or estrogen/progestin regimens on heart disease risk factors in postmenopausal women. The Postmenopausal Estrogen/Progestin Interventions (PEPI) Trial. The Writing Group for the PEPI Trial." *JAMA.* 1995; 273:199–208.

Furberg, C.D. *et al.* "Subgroup interactions in the Heart and Estrogen/Progestin Replacement Study: lessons learned." *Circulation.* 2002; 105:917–922.

Grady, D. *et al.* "Cardiovascular disease outcomes during 6.8 years of hormone therapy: Heart and Estrogen/progestin Replacement Study follow-up (HERS II)." *JAMA.* 2002; 288:49–57.

Grady, D. *et al.* "Hormone therapy to prevent disease and prolong life in postmenopausal women." *Ann Intern Med.* 1992; 117:1016–1037.

"Guidelines for counseling postmenopausal women about preventive hormone therapy." American College of Physicians. *Ann Intern Med.* 1992; 117:1038-1041.

Hemminki, E., and K. McPherson. "Impact of postmenopausal hormone therapy on cardiovascular events and cancer: pooled data from clinical trials." *BMJ.* 1997; 315:149-153.

Hemminki, E., and K. McPherson. "Value of drug-licensing documents in studying the effect of postmenopausal hormone therapy on cardiovascular disease." *Lancet.* 2000; 355:566-569.

Herrington, D.M. *et al.* "Comparison of the Heart and Estrogen/Progestin Replacement Study (HERS) cohort with women with coronary disease from the National Health and Nutrition Examination Survey III (NHANES III)." *Am Heart J.* 1998; 136:115-124.

Herrington, D.M. *et al.* "Effects of estrogen replacement on the progression of coronary-artery atherosclerosis." *N Engl J Med.* 2000; 343:522-529.

Hodis, H.N. *et al.* "Estrogen in the prevention of atherosclerosis. A randomized, double-blind, placebo-controlled trial." *Ann Intern Med.* 2001; 135:939-953.

Horwitz, R.I. *et al.* "Treatment adherence and risk of death after a myocardial infarction." *Lancet.* 1990; 336:542-545.

Hsia, J. *et al.* "Peripheral arterial disease in randomized trial of estrogen with progestin in women with coronary heart disease: the Heart and Estrogen / Progestin Replacement Study." *Circulation.* 2000; 102:2228-2232.

Hu, F.B. *et al.* "Age at natural menopause and risk of cardiovascular disease." *Arch Intern Med.* 1999; 159:1061-1066.

Hulley, S. *et al.* "Randomized trial of estrogen plus progestin for secondary prevention of coronary heart disease in postmenopausal women. Heart and Estrogen/ progestin Replacement Study (HERS) Research Group." *JAMA.* 1998; 280:605-613.

Humphrey, L.L. *et al.* "Postmenopausal hormone replacement therapy and the primary prevention of cardiovascular disease." *Ann Intern Med.* 2002; 137:273-284.

Iribarren, C. *et al.* "Twelve-year trends in cardiovascular disease risk factors in the Minnesota Heart Survey. Are socioeconomic differences widening?" *Arch Intern Med.* 1997; 157:873-881.

Isles, C.G. *et al.* "Relation between coronary risk and coronary mortality in women of the Renfrew and Paisley survey: comparison with men." *Lancet.* 1992; 339:702-706.

Jacobs, D.R., Jr. *et al.* "High density lipoprotein cholesterol as a predictor of cardiovascular disease mortality in men and women: the follow-up study of the Lipid Research Clinics Prevalence Study." *Am J Epidemiol.* 1990; 131:32-47.

Jayachandran, M., and V.M. Miller. "Molecular and cellular mechanisms of estrogen's actions." In: Douglas, P.S., ed. *Cardiovascular Health and Disease in Women.* 2nd ed. 2002; Philadelphia: WB Saunders;207-230.

Kalin, M.F., and B. Zumoff. "Sex hormones and coronary disease: a review of the clinical studies." *Steroids.* 1990; 55:330-352.

Key, T. et al. "Endogenous sex hormones and breast cancer in postmenopausal women: reanalysis of nine prospective studies." *J Natl Cancer Inst.* 2002; 94:606–616.

Lenfant, C. National Heart, Lung, and Blood Institute Communications Office, Press Release, April 3, 2000.

Matthews, K.A. et al. "Prior to use of estrogen replacement therapy, are users healthier than nonusers?" *Am J Epidemiol.* 1996; 143:971–978.

Mendelsohn, M.E., and R.H. Karas. "The protective effects of estrogen on the cardiovascular system." *N Engl J Med.* 1999; 340:1801–1811.

Michels, K.B., and J.E. Manson. "Postmenopausal hormone therapy: a reversal of fortune." *Circulation.* 2003; 107:1830–1833.

Mikkola, T.S., and T.B. Clarkson. "Estrogen replacement therapy, atherosclerosis, and vascular function." *Cardiovasc Res.* 2002;53: 605–619.

"Mild Thyroid Failure and High Cholesterol May Go Hand in Hand." American Thyroid Association, Press Release. Sept 17, 2003.

Osler, W. "Lectures on angina pectoris and allied states." *NY Med J.* 1896; 64:20–44.

Passino, C. et al. "Aerobic Training Decreases B-Type Natriuretic Peptide Expression and Adrenergic Activation in Patients With Heart Failure." *Journal of the American College of Cardiology.* 2006; 47(9):1835-1839.

Petitti, D.B. "Coronary heart disease and estrogen replacement therapy. Can compliance bias explain the results of observational studies?" *Ann Epidemiol.* 1994; 4:115–118.

Piepoli, M.F. et al. "Exercise training meta-analysis of trials in patients with chronic heart failure (ExTraMATCH)." *BMJ.* 2004 Jan 24; 328(7433):189. Epub 2004 Jan 16.

Posthuma, W.F. et al. "Cardioprotective effect of hormone replacement therapy in postmenopausal women: is the evidence biased?" *BMJ.* 1994; 308:1268–1269.

Psaty, B.M. et al. "Hormone replacement therapy, prothrombotic mutations, and the risk of incident nonfatal myocardial infarction in postmenopausal women." *JAMA.* 2001; 285:906–913.

"Research on the menopause in the 1990s: report of a World Health Organization Scientific Group." Geneva: World Health Organization Tech Rep Ser. 1996; No 866:0512–3054.

Rossouw, J.E. et al. "Risks and benefits of estrogen plus progestin in healthy postmenopausal women: principal results from the Women's Health Initiative randomized controlled trial." *JAMA.* 2002; 288:321–333.

Shapiro, S. "Meta-analysis/Shmeta-analysis." *Am J Epidemiol.* 1994; 140:771–778.

Simon, J.A. et al. "Postmenopausal hormone therapy and risk of stroke: The Heart and Estrogen-progestin Replacement Study (HERS)." *Circulation.* 2001;103: 638–642.

Stampfer, M.J., and G.A. Colditz. "Estrogen replacement therapy and coronary heart disease: a quantitative assessment of the epidemiologic evidence." *Prev Med.* 1991; 20:47–63.

"The Coronary Drug Project. Initial findings leading to modifications of its research protocol." *JAMA.* 1970; 214:1303–1313.

"The Coronary Drug Project. Findings leading to discontinuation of the 2.5-mg day estrogen group. The Coronary Drug Project Research Group." *JAMA.* 1973; 226:652–657.

Tikkanen, M.J. *et al.* "High density lipoprotein-2 and hepatic lipase: reciprocal changes produced by estrogen and norgestrel." *J Clin Endocrinol Metab.* 1982; 54:1113–1117.

Tracy, R.E. "Sex difference in coronary disease: two opposing views." *J Chronic Dis.* 1966;19: 1245–1251.

U.S. Preventive Services Task Force. Guide to Clinical Preventive Services, 3rd ed, 2000–2003. Chemoprevention: hormone replacement therapy. (www.ahcpr.gov/clinic/3rduspstf/hrt/hrtrr.htm.)

Van der Schouw, Y.T. *et al.* "Age at menopause as a risk factor for cardiovascular mortality." *Lancet.* 1996; 347:714–718.

Vandenbroucke, J.P. "Postmenopausal oestrogen and cardioprotection." *Lancet.* 1991; 337:1482–1483.

Visser, M. *et al.* "Elevated C-Reactive Protein Levels in Overweight and Obese Adults." *JAMA.* 1999; 282:2131-2135.

Walsh, B.W. *et al.* "The effects of hormone replacement therapy and raloxifene on C-reactive protein and homocysteine in healthy postmenopausal women: a randomized, controlled trial." *J Clin Endocrinol Metab.* 2000; 85:214–218.

Waters, D.D. *et al.* "Effects of hormone replacement therapy and antioxidant vitamin supplements on coronary atherosclerosis in postmenopausal women: a randomized controlled trial." *JAMA.* 2002; 288:2432–2440.

Wenger, N.K. *et al.* "Early risks of hormone therapy in patients with coronary heart disease." *JAMA.* 2000;284: 41–43.

"WHI Steering Committee and Writing Group Response, Letter to the Editor." *JAMA.* 2002; 288: 2823–2824.

Wilson, P.W. *et al.* "Postmenopausal estrogen use, cigarette smoking, and cardiovascular morbidity in women over 50. The Framingham Study." *N Engl J Med.* 1985; 313:1038–1043.

Yusuf, S. *et al.* "Obesity and the risk of myocardial infarction in 27,000 participants from 52 countries, a case-controlled study." *Lancet.* 2005; 366:1640-1649.

The Lowdown on Cholesterol and High Blood Pressure

Aono, Y. *et al.* "Plasma Fibrinogen, Ambulatory Blood Pressure, and Silent Cerebrovascular Lesions: The Ohasama Study." *Arterioscler Thromb Vasc Biol.* 2007 Apr; 27(4):963-8.

Blood Pressure Statistics, Heart and Stroke Foundation of Canada (www.heartandstroke.com) and American Heart Foundation (www.americanheart.org).

Clays, E. *et al.* "Associations Between Dimensions of Job Stress and Biomarkers of Inflammation and Infection." *J Occup and Env Med.* 2005; 47(9):878-883.

Coppola, G. *et al.* "Fibrinogen as a predictor of mortality after acute myocardial infarction: a forty-two-month follow-up study." *Ital Heart J.* 2005 Apr; 6(4):315-22.

Danesh, J. *et al.* "Lipoprotein(a) and Coronary Heart Disease." *Circulation.* 2000; 102:1082.

Danesh, J. *et al.* "Plasma Fibrinogen Level and the Risk of Major Cardiovascular Diseases and Nonvascular Mortality: An Individual Participant Meta-analysis." *JAMA.* 2005; 294(14):1799-809.

Ferritin Testing Ranges, U.S. National Institutes of Health Medline Plus (www.nlm.nih.gov/medlineplus/).

Fibrinogen Testing Ranges, U.S. National Institutes of Health Medline Plus, (www.nlm.nih.gov/medlineplus/).

Graham, I.M. *et al.* "Plasma Homocysteine as a Risk Factor for Vascular Disease." *JAMA.* 1997; 277(22):1775-1781.

Lipoprotein A and Apolipoprotein B Levels, U.S. National Institutes of Health, Medline Plus (www.nlm.nih.gov/medlineplus/) and J. Jacques Genest et al. "Recommendations for the Management of Dyslipidemia and the Prevention of Cardiovascular Disease: 2003 Update." *CMAJ.* 2003; 168(9):921-4.

Malinow, M.R. *et al.* "Homocyst(e)ine, Diet, and Cardiovascular Diseases: A Statement for Healthcare Professionals from the Nutrition Committee, American Heart Association." *Circulation.* 1999; 99:178-82.

Metamatrix Clinical Laboratories Cardiovascular Health Profile Testing, (www.metametrix.com/DirectoryOfServices/pdf/pdf_sample_0161CardiovascularHealth-Blood.pdf)

National Heart, Lung and Blood Institute's National Cholesterol Education Program Cholesterol Level Recommendations, 2001.

Recommended Triglyceride Levels for the U.S. and Canada, The Mayo Clinic (www.mayoclinic.com).

Ridker, P.M. *et al.* "Inflammation, Aspirin, and the Risk of Cardiovascular Disease in Apparently Healthy Men." *N Engl J Med.* 1997; 336(14):973-9.

Ridker, P.M. *et al.* "Prospective Study of C-reactive Protein and the Risk of Future Cardiovascular Events Among Apparently Healthy Women." *Circulation.* 1998; 98(8):731-3.

Robinson, K. *et al.* "Hyperhomocysteinemia and Low Pyridoxal Phosphate. Common and Independent Reversible Risk Factors for Coronary Artery Disease." *Circulation.* 1995; 92(10):2825-30.

Sachdeva, A. *et al.* "Lipid Levels in Patients Hospitalized with Coronary Artery Disease: An Analysis of 136,905 Hospitalizations in *Get With The Guidelines.*" *Am Heart J.* 2009; 157(1):111-117.e2.

Whincup, P. *et al.* "Serum total homocysteine and coronary heart disease: prospective study in middle aged men." *Heart.* 1999; 82(4):448–454.

Xilin, Y. *et al.* "Independent Associations Between Low-density Lipoprotein Cholesterol and Cancer Among Patients with Type 2 Diabetes Mellitus." *CMAJ.* 2008; 179(5):427-37.

Zoccali, C. *et al.* "Fibrinogen, mortality and incident cardiovascular complications in end-stage renal failure." *J Intern Med.* 2003; 254(2):132-9.

Diabetes and Depression: Double Trouble

Bunker, S.J. *et al.* " 'Stress' and Coronary Heart Disease: Psychosocial Risk Factors." *Med J Aust.* 2003; 178(6):272-6.

"Can Pets Help Keep You Healthy? Exploring the Human-Animal Bond." *NIH News in Health*, National Institutes of Health, February 2009, eNewsletter.

Centers for Disease Control, National Diabetes Fact Sheet 2007 (www.cdc.gov/diabetes/pubs/pdf/ndfs_2007.pdf).

Depression Symptoms, the College of Family Physicians of Canada, www.cfpa.ca (www.healthywomen.org/Documents/NationalWomensHealthReport.August2003.pdf)

Diabetes-Heart Disease Connection, American Diabetes Association, (www.diabetes.org/heart-disease-stroke.jsp)

Diabetes Prevention Program Research Group. "Effect of Progression From Impaired Glucose Tolerance to Diabetes on Cardiovascular Risk Factors and Its Amelioration by Lifestyle and Metformin Intervention" Diabetes Care. 2009; 32(4):726-732

Diabetes Prevention Program Research Group "Reduction in the Incidence of Type 2 Diabetes with Lifestyle Intervention or Metformin." *NEJM.* 2002; 346(6):393-403.

Glucose Tolerance Testing, National Institutes of Health Medline Plus, (www.nlm.nih.gov/medlineplus/ency/article/003466.htm)

Khaw, K. *et al.* "Glycated Haemoglobin, Diabetes, and Mortality in Men in Norfolk Cohort of European Prospective Investigation of Cancer and Nutrition (EPIC-Norfolk)." *BMJ* 2001; 322:15.

McGrath, E. *et al.* "Women and Depression: Risk Factors and Treatment Issues." 1990. Washington, DC: American Psychological Association.

Mittleman, M.A. *et al.* "Triggering of Acute Myocardial Infarction Onset by Episodes of Anger." *Circulation.* 1995; 92:1720-1725.

Penninx, B.W. *et al.* "Depression and Cardiac Mortality: Results from a Community based Longitudinal Study." *Arch Gen Psychiatry.* 2001; 58(3):221-7.

Ratner, R.E. *et al.* "Prevention of Diabetes in Women with a History of Gestational Diabetes: Effects of Metformin and Lifestyle Interventions." *J Clin Endocrinol Metab.* 2008; 93(12):4774-4779.

Reed, D. *et al.* "Social Networks and Coronary Heart Disease among Japanese Men in Hawaii." *Am J Epidemiol.* 1983 Apr; 117(4):384-96.

Wellenius, G.A. *et al.* "Depressive Symptoms and the Risk of Atherosclerotic Progression Among Patients With Coronary Artery Bypass Grafts." *Circulation.* 2008; 117:2313-2319.

Whang, W. *et al.* "Depression and Risk of Sudden Cardiac Death and Coronary Heart Disease in Women." *J Am Coll Cardiol.* 2009; 53:950-958.

Yoichi, C., and A. Steptoe. "The Association of Anger and Hostility with Future Coronary Heart Disease: A Meta-Analytic Review of Prospective Evidence." *J Am Coll Cardiol.* 2009; 53:936-946.

Heart-Smarten Up on Carbs and Fats

Ascherio, A. *et al.* "Dietary Fat and Risk of Coronary Heart Disease in Men: Cohort Follow up Study in the United States." *BMJ.* 1996; 313(7049):84-90.

Assuncao, M.L. *et al.* "Effects of Dietary Coconut Oil on the Biochemical and Anthropometric Profiles of Women Presenting Abdominal Obesity." *Lipids.* 2009 May 13; [Epub ahead of print].

Djousse, L. *et al.* "Relation Between Dietary Linolenic acid and Coronary Artery Disease in the National Heart, Lung and Blood Institute Family Heart Study. *Am J Clin Nutr.* 2001; 74:612-619.

Gillum, R.F. *et al.* "The Relationship Between Fish Consumption and Stroke Incidence: The NHANES I Epidemiologic Follow-up Study (National Health and Nutrition Examination Survey). *Arch Intern Med.* 1996; 156:537-542.

Holub, B.J. "Docosahexaenoic Acid (DHA) and Cardiovascular Disease Risk Factors." Prostaglandins Leukot Essent Fatty Acids. 2009 Jun 20. [Epub ahead of print].

Hu, F.B. *et al.* "Fish and Omega-3 Fatty Acid Intake and Risk of Coronary Heart Disease in Women." *JAMA.* 2002; 287:1815-1821.

Iso, H. *et al.* "Intake of Fish and Omega-3 Fatty Acids and Risk of Stroke in Women." *JAMA.* 2001; 285:304-312.

James, M.J. *et al.* "Metabolism of Stearidonic Acid in Human Subjects: Comparison with the Metabolism of Other n-3 Fatty Acids." *Am J Clin Nutr.* 2003; 77(5):1140-5.

Laaksonen, D.E. *et al.* "Prediction of Cardiovascular Mortality in Middle-aged Men by Dietary and Serum Linoleic and Polyunsaturated Fatty Acids." *Arch Intern Med.* 2005; 165(2):193-199.

Mozaffarian, D. "Fish and n-3 Fatty Acids for the Prevention of Fatal Coronary Heart Disease and Sudden Cardiac Death." *Am J Clin Nutr.* 2008; 87(6):1991S-1996S.

Oh, K. *et al.* "Dietary Fat Intake and Risk of Coronary Heart Disease in Women: 20 Years of Follow-up of the Nurses' Health Study." *Am J Epidemiol.* 2005; 161(7):672-679.

Shekelle, R.B. *et al.* "Diet, Serum Cholesterol, and Death from Coronary Heart Disease. The Western Electric Study." *NEJM.* 1981; 304(2):65-70.

Sircus, M. OMD. Magnesium: The Ultimate Heart Medicine. eBook, 2009. (www.imva.info)

Siscovick, D.S. *et al.* "Dietary Intake and Cell Membrane Levels of Long-chain n-3 Polyunsaturated Fatty Acids and the Risk of Primary Cardiac Arrest." *JAMA.* 1995; 274:1363-1367.

Stone, N.J. "Fish Consumption, Fish Oil, Lipids, and Coronary Heart Disease." *Circulation.* 1996; 94:2337-2340.

Surette, M.E. *et al.* "Dietary Echium Oil Increases Plasma and Neutrophil Long-Chain (n-3) Fatty Acids and Lowers Serum Triacylglycerols in Hypertriglyceridemic Humans." *American Society for Nutritional Sciences J. Nutr.* 2004 June; 134:1406-1411.

Zhang, P. *et al.* "Echium Oil Reduces Plasma Lipids and Hepatic Lipogenic Gene

Expression in ApoB100-only LDL Receptor Knockout Mice." *J Nutr Biochem.* 2008; 19(10):655-63. Epub 2007 Dec 21.

Eat the Heart Healthy Way

Almoznino-Sarafian, D. *et al.* "Magnesium Administration May Improve Heart Rate Variability in Patients with Heart Failure." *Nutr Metab Cardiovasc Dis.* 2009 Feb 6; [Epub ahead of print].

Almoznino-Sarafian, D. *et al.* "Magnesium and C-reactive Protein in Heart Failure: An Anti-inflammatory Effect of Magnesium Administration?" *Eur J Nutr.* 2007; 46(4):230-237.

Aviram, M. *et al.* "Pomegranate Juice Consumption for 3 Years by Patients with Carotid Artery Stenosis Reduces Common Carotid Intima-media Thickness, Blood Pressure and LDL Oxidation." *Clin Nutr.* 2004; 23(3):423-33.

Aviram, M. *et al.* "Pomegranate Juice Flavonoids Inhibit Low-density Lipoprotein Oxidation and Cardiovascular Diseases: Studies in Atherosclerotic Mice and Humans." Drugs Under Experimental and Clinical Research. 2002; XXVIII (2-3):49-62.

Debette, S. *et al.* "Tea Consumption Is Inversely Associated With Carotid Plaques in Women." *Atheroslcerosis, Thrombosis, and Vascular Biology.* 2008; 28(2):353-359.

Dedoussis, G.V. *et al.* "Mediterranean Diet and Plasma Concentration of Inflammatory Markers in Old and Very Old Subjects in the ZINCAGE Population Study." *Clin Chem Lab Med.* 2008; 46(7): 990-996.

Fito, M. *et al.* "Effect of a Traditional Mediterranean Diet on Lipoprotein Oxidation: A Randomized Controlled Trial." *Arch Intern Med.* 2007; 167(11):1195-1203.

Food Charts for Potassium and Magnesium, Sources: USDA Nutrient Database for Standard References; Canadian Nutrient File, 2007b, Health Canada.

Fuhrman, B. *et al.* "Pomegranate Juice Inhibits Oxidized LDL Uptake and Cholesterol Biosynthesis in Macrophages." *J Nutr Biochem.* 2005; 16(9):570-6.

Fung, T.T. *et al.* "Sweetened Beverage Consumption and Risk of Coronary Heart Disease in Women." *Am J Clin Nutr.* 2009; 89(4):1037-42.

Galeone, C. *et al.* "Allium vegetable intake and risk of acute myocardial infarction in Italy." *Eur J Nutr.* 2009; 48(2):120-3.

Gardner, E.J. *et al.* "Black tea—helpful or harmful? A Review of the Evidence." *Eur J Clin Nutr.* 2007; 61(1):3-18.

Geleijnse, J.M. *et al.* "Dietary Intake of Menaquinone Is Associated with a Reduced Risk of Coronary Heart Disease: The Rotterdam Study." *J. Nutr.* 2004; 134:3100-3105.

Halton, T.L. *et al.* "Low-carbohydrate-diet score and the risk of coronary heart disease in women." *NEJM.* 2006; 355(19):1991-2002.

Huang, T.H. *et al.* "Anti-diabetic Action of Punica Granatum Flower Extract: Activation of PPAR-gamma and Identification of an Active Component. *Toxicol Appl Pharmacol.* 2005; 207(2):160-9.

Kaplan, M. *et al.* "Pomegranate Juice Supplementation to Atherosclerotic Mice Reduces Macrophage Lipid Peroxidation, Cellular Cholesterol Accumulation and Development of Atherosclerosis." *Biochemical and Molecular Action of Nutrients.* 2001; 131(8):2082-9.

Kris-Etherton, P. et al. "Lyon Diet Heart Study Benefits of a Mediterranean-Style, National Cholesterol Education Program/American Heart Association Step I Dietary Pattern on Cardiovascular Disease." *Circulation*. 2001; 103:1823.

Mente, A. et al. "A Systematic Review of the Evidence Supporting a Causal Link Between Dietary Factors and Coronary Heart Disease" *Arch Intern Med*. 2009; 169(7):659-66.

Miller, S. et al. "Effects of Magnesium on Atrial Fibrillation After Cardiac Surgery: A Meta-Analysis." *Heart*. 2005; 91:618-623.

Mozaffari-Khosravi, H. et al. "The Effects of Sour Tea (Hibiscus Sabdariffa) on Hypertension in Patients with Type II Diabetes." *J Hum Hypertens*. 2009; 23(1):48-54.

Nunez-Cordoba, J.M. et al. "The Mediterranean Diet and Incidence of Hypertension: The Seguimiento Universidad de Navarra (SUN) Study." *Am J Epidemiol*. 2009; 169(3):339-46.

Rosanoff, A., and M.S. Seelig. "Comparison of Mechanism and Functional Effects of Magnesium and Statin Pharmaceuticals." *J Am Coll Nutr*. 2004; 23(5):501S-505S.

Sacks, F.M. et al. "Effects on Blood Pressure of Reduced Dietary Sodium and the Dietary Approaches to Stop Hypertension (DASH) Diet. DASH-Sodium Collaborative Research Group." *N Engl J Med*. 2001; 344(1): 3-10.

Sanchez-Tainta, A. et al. "Adherence to a Mediterranean-type Diet and Reduced Prevalence of Clustered Cardiovascular Risk Factors in a Cohort of 3204 High-risk Patients." *Eur J Cardiovasc Prev Rehabil*. 2008; 15(5):589-593.

Sastravaha, G. et al. "Adjunctive Periodontal Treatment with Centella asiatica and Punica granatum Extracts in Supportive Periodontal Therapy." *J Int Acad Periodontol*. 2005; 7(3):70-9.

Shechter, M. et al. "Effects of Oral Magnesium Therapy on Exercise Tolerance, Exercise-Induced Chest Pain, and Quality of Life in Patients with Coronary Artery Disease." *Am J Cardiol*. 2003; 91:517-521.

Shechter, M. et al. "Magnesium Therapy in Acute Myocardial Infarction When Patients Are not Candidates for Thrombolytic Therapy." *Am J Cardiol*. 1995; 75(5): 321-323.

Schurgers, L.J. et al. "Vitamin K-containing dietary supplements: comparison of synthetic vitamin K1 and natto-derived menaquinone-7." *Blood*. 2007; 109(8):3279-83.

Sepura, O.B., and A.I. Martynow. "Magnesium Orotate in Severe Congestive Heart Failure (MACH)." *Int J Cardiol*. 2009; 134(1):145-7.

Sumner, M.D. et al. "Effects of Pomegranate Juice Consumption on Myocardial Perfusion in Patients with Coronary Heart Disease." *Am J Cardiol*. 2005; 96(6):810-4.

Umesawa, M. et al. "Sodium, Potassium, Diet Reference: "Relations Between Dietary Sodium and Potassium Intakes and Mortality from Cardiovascular Disease: The Japan Collaborative Cohort Study for Evaluation of Cancer Risks." *Am J Clin Nutr*. 2008; 88(1):195-202.

Heart Health Nutrients

Araghi-Niknam, M. *et al.* "Pine bark extract reduces platelet aggregation." *Integr Med.* 2000; 2(2): 73-77.

Belcaro, G. *et al.* "Prevention of venous thrombophlebitis in long-haul flights with Pycnogenol." *Clin Appl Thromb Hemost.* 2004; 10 (4):373-377.

Buzzard, A.R. *et al.* "Kyolic and Pycnogenol increases human growth hormone secretion in genetically-engineered keratinocytes." *Growth Hormone & IGF Research.* 2002; 12, 34-40.

Canner, P.L. *et al.* "Fifteen Year Mortality in Coronary Drug Project Patients: Long-term Benefit with Niacin." *J Am Coll Cardiol.* 1986; 8:1245-1255.

Cesarone, M.R. *et al.* "Prevention of edema in long flights with pycnogenol." *Clin Appl Thromb Hemost.* 2005; 11(3):289-294.

Cupp, M.J., and T.S. Tracy, eds. "Chapter 4: Coenzyme Q10 (Ubiquinone, Ubidecarenone)." *Dietary Supplements,* Humana Press; Totowa (New Jersey), 2003, 53-85.

Dilman, V., and W. Dean. *The Neuroendocrine Theory of Aging and Degenerative Disease.* The Center for Bio-Gerontology, Pensacola, 1992.

Fitzpatrick, D.F. *et al.* "Endothelium-dependent vascular effects of pycnogenol." *J Cardiovasc Pharmacol.* 1998; 32:509-515.

Gulati, O.P. "Pycnogenol in venous disorders: A review." *Eur Bull Drug Res.* 1999; 7(2):8-13.

Guyton, J.R. *et al.* "Extended-release Niacin vs. Gemfibrozil for the Treatment of Low Levels of High Density Lipoprotein Cholesterol." *Arch Intern Med.* 2000; 160:1177-1184.

Hasegawa, N. "Inhibition of lipogenesis by pycnogenol." *Phytother Res.* 2000; 14(6):472-473.

Hasegawa, N. "Stimulation of lipolysis by pycnogenol." *Phytother Res.* 1999; 13 (7),619-620.

Horowitz, N. "Link Niacin to Longevity after an MI." *Medical Tribune.* 1985, 26(12):1, 17.

Hosseini, S. *et al.* "A randomized, double blind, placebo controlled, prospective, 16 week crossover study to determine the role of Pycnogenol in modifying blood pressure in mildly hypertensive patients." *Nutr Res.* 2001; 21(9):67-76.

Hosseini, S. *et al.* "Pycnogenol in the management of asthma." *Journal of Medicinal Food.* 2001b; 4(4): 201-209.

Kohana, T., and N. Suzuki. "The treatment of gynaecological disorders with Pycnogenol." *Eur Bull Drug Res.* 1999; 7:30-32.

Liu, X. *et al.* "Antidiabetic effect of Pycnogenol French maritime pine bark extract in patients with diabetes type II." *Life Sci.* 2004b; 75(21):2505-2513.

Liu, X. *et al.* "Pycnogenol, French maritime pine bark extract, improves endothelial function of hypertensive patients." *Life Sci.* 2004a; 74(7):855-862.

Mochizuki, M., and N. Hasegawa. "Pycnogenol stimulates lipolysis in 3t3-L1 cells via stimulation of beta-receptor mediated activity." *Phytother Res.* 2004; 18(12):1029-1030.

Mohaupt, M.G. *et al.* "Association between statin-associated myopathy and skeletal muscle damage." *CMAJ.* 2009; 181(1-2). [Epub ahead of print.]

Nelson, A.B. *et al.* "Pycnogenol inhibits macrophage oxidative burst, lipoprotein oxidation, and hydroxyl radical-induced DNA damage." *Drug Dev Ind Pharm.* 1998; 24 (2):139-144.

Ohira, T. "Serum and Dietary Magnesium and Risk of Ischemic Stroke: The Atherosclerosis Risk in Communities Study." *Am J Epidemiol.* 2009; 169(12):1437-1444.

Packer, L. *et al.* "Antioxidant activity and biologic properties of a procyanidin-rich extract from Pine (Pinus maritime) bark, Pycnogenol." *Free Radical Biology and Medicine.* 1999; 27(5/6):704-724.

Pavlovic, P. "Improved endurance by use of antioxidants. *Eur Bull Drug Res.* 1999; 7(2):26-29.

Peng, Q. *et al.* "Pycnogenol inhibits tumour necrosis factor-alpha-induced nuclear factor kappa B activation and adhesion molecule expression in human vascular endothelial cells." *Cell Mol Life Sci.* 2000; 57(5):834-841.

Pocobelli, G. *et al.* "Use of Supplements of Multivitamins, Vitamin C and Vitamin E in Relation to Mortality." *Am J Epidemiol.* 2009; 170(4):472-83. Epub 2009 Jul 13.

Putter, M. *et al.* "Inhibition of smoking-induced platelet aggregation by aspirin and pycnogenol." *Thromb Res.* 1999; 95(4):155-161.

Quereshi, A. *et al.* "Response of Hypercholesterolemic Subjects to Administration of Tocotrienols. *Lipid.* 1995; 30:1171-1177.

Rihn, B. *et al.* "From ancient remedies to modern therapeutics: Pine bark uses in skin disorders revisited." *Phytother Res.* 2001; 15:76-78.

Roseff, S.J. "Improvement in sperm quality and function with French maritime pine tree bark extract." *J Reprod Med.* 2000; 47(10):821-824.

Rosenfeldt, F.L. *et al.* "Coenzyme Q10 in the Treatment of Hypertension: A Meta-analysis of the Clinical Trials." *J Human Hypertension.* 2007; 21:297-306.

Saliou, C. *et al.* "Solar ultraviolet-induced erythema in human skin and nuclear factor-kappa-B-dependent gene expression in keratinocytes are modulated by a French maritime pine bark extract." *Free Rad Biol Med.* 2001; 30(2):154-160.

Simme, S., and V.E. Reeve. "Protection from inflammation, immunosuppression and carcinogenesis induced by UV radiation in mice by topical Pycnogenol." *Photochem Photobiol.* 2004; 79(2):193-198.

Talbott, S.M. *et al.* "Effect of Citrus Flavonoids and Tocotrienols on Serum Cholesterol Levels in Hypercholesterolemic Subjects." *Altern Ther Health Med.* 2007; 13(6):44-8.

Tixier, J.M. *et al.* "Evidence by in vivo and in vitro studies that binding of Pycnogenol to elastin affects its rate of degradation by elastase." *Biochem Pharmacol.* 1984; 33; 3933-3939.

Vina, J. *et al.* "Free radicals in exhaustive physical exercise: mechanism of production and protection by antioxidants." *Life.* 2000; 50(4-5):271-277.

Wei, Z. *et al.* "Pycnogenol enhances endothelial cell antioxidant defences." *Redox Rep.* 1997; 3: 147-155.

Heart Health Fitness

Albright, C., and D.L. Thompson. "The Effectiveness of Walking in Preventing Cardiovascular Disease in Women: A Review of the Current Literature." *Journal of Women's Health*. 2006; 15(3): 271-280.

Blumenthal, J.A. *et al.* "Effects of Exercise and Stress Management Training on Markers of Cardiovascular Risk in Patients With Ischemic Heart Disease" *JAMA*. 2005; 293:1626-1634.

Gordon-Larsen, P. *et al.* "Active Commuting and Cardiovascular Disease Risk The CARDIA Study." *Arch Intern Med*. 2009; 169(13):1216-1223

Rothenbacher, D. *et al.* "Lifetime physical activity patterns and risk of coronary heart disease." *Heart*. 2006; 92:1319-1320.

"Sudden Exercise Poses Risk" BBC News, December 31, 2003.

How to Tame Stress

Bertisch, S.M. *et al.* "Alternative Mind-body Therapies Used by Adults with Medical Conditions." *J Psychosom Res*. 2009; 66(6):511-9.

Carlson, L.E. *et al.* "One Year Pre-post Intervention Follow-up of Psychological, Immune, Endocrine and Blood Pressure Outcomes of Mindfulness-based Stress Reduction (MBSR) in Breast and Prostate Cancer Outpatients." *Brain Behav Immun*. 2007; 21(8):1038-49.

Chaya, M.S. *et al.* "Insulin Sensitivity and Cardiac Autonomic Function in Young Male Practitioners of Yoga." *Natl Med J India*. 2008; 21(5):217-21.

Hadj, A. *et al.* "Pre-operative preparation for cardiac surgery utilising a combination of metabolic, physical and mental therapy." *Heart Lung Circ*. 2006; 15(3):172-81. Epub 2006 May 19.

Holman, E.A. *et al.* "Terrorism, Acute Stress, and Cardiovascular Health." *Arch Gen Psychiatry*. 2008; 65(1):73-80.

Jancin, B. "Yoga Helps Endothelial Function in Heart Patients." *Family Practice News*. 2004 December 15: 12.

Manikonda, J.P. *et al.* "Contemplative Meditation Reduces Ambulatory Blood Pressure and Stress-induced Hypertension: A Randomized Pilot Trial." *J Hum Hypertens*. 2008; 22(2):138-40.

Paul-Labrador, M. *et al.* "Effects of a Randomized Controlled Trial of Transcendental Meditation on Components of the Metabolic Syndrome in Subjects with Coronary Heart Disease." *Arch Intern Med*. 2006; 166(11):1218-24.

Pullen, P.R. *et al.* "Effects of Yoga on Inflammation and Exercise Capacity in Patients with Chronic Heart Failure." *J Card Fail*. 2008; 14(5):407-13.

Sivasankaran, S. "The Effect of a Six-week Program of Yoga and Meditation on Brachial Artery Reactivity: Do Psychosocial Interventions Affect Vascular Tone?" *Clin Cardiol*. 2006; 29(9):393-8.

Sullivan, M.J. *et al.* "The Support, Education, and Research in Chronic Heart Failure Study (SEARCH): A Mindfulness-based Psychoeducational Intervention Improves Depression and Clinical Symptoms in Patients with Chronic Heart Failure." *Am Heart J*. 2009; 157(1):84-90.

Think Happy, Live with Heart

Eremin, O. *et al*. "Immuno-modulatory Effects of Relaxation Training and Guided Imagery in Women with Locally Advanced Breast Cancer Undergoing Multimodality Therapy: A Randomised Controlled Trial." *Breast*. 2009; 18(1):17-25.

Jancin, B. "Pleasurable Lifestyle Changes Can Cut Cardiac Risk." *Family Practice News*. 1998 December 15: 14-15.

Liu, K.P. *et al*. "A Randomized Controlled Trial of Mental Imagery Augment Generalization of Learning in Acute Poststroke Patients." *Stroke*. 2009 Jun; 40(6):2222-5.

Miller, M., and W.F. Fry. "The Effect of Mirthful Laughter on the Human Cardiovascular System." *Med Hypotheses*. 2009 May 26. [Epub ahead of print]

"University of Maryland School of Medicine Study Shows Laughter Helps Blood Vessels Function Better." University of Maryland, Media Release, March 7, 2005.

Index

A

adrenal glands, 57-59
age, 19-20
alcohol consumption, 97
amino acids, 87-88
anger, 63-65
angina, 13-14
  and Coenzyme Q10, 177
antioxidants, 12-13
anxiety, 65-66
apolipoprotein B (Apo B), 43
arrhythmia, 14
arteries, 8, 9
arteriosclerosis vs.
  atherosclerosis, 8
artificial sweeteners, 111
Ascherio, Alberto, 77
aspirin, 178
assessment of heart health, 105-8
atherosclerosis, 6, 13
  vs. arteriosclerosis, 8
avocado, 123

B

bioidentical progesterone, 27, 28
birth control pills see oral
  contraceptives
blood clots, 13
  and fibrinogen, 45-46
  and pycnogenol, 174
blood flow to heart, 8-9, 15
blood pressure see high blood
  pressure (hypertension)
body mass index (BMI), 35-36
body shape, 38
bone health (postmenopausal), 31
breathing, deep, 224-27
butter, 75

C

C-reactive protein (CRP), 47-49
caffeine, 97-98
calcification, 92-93
calcium and magnesium, 29-32
carbohydrates, 67-72, 87
cardiovascular disease, 2, 6-7
  and calcium and magnesium, 29-32
cardiovascular tests, 49
Chek, Paul, 192
Chlamydia pneumoniae, 48
cholesterol, 9-11, 39-40
  cholesterol levels, 40-42
  dietary vs. blood, 11
  high-density lipoprotein (HDL), 10, 41
  low-density lipoprotein (LDL), 10,
    11, 41-42
  and magnesium, 180-81
  and niacin, 183-85
  and sytrinol, 166-70, 172
  very low-density lipoproteins
    (VLDL), 39, 40, 42
coconut oil, 75-76
Coenzyme Q10, 175-79
coffee, 97-98
cognitive loss (postmenopausal), 31
cooking tips, 113, 114
  flax meal, 114
  food processors, 114
  grains, 110, 116
  low-heat sautéing, 112
  oils, 113, 114-15
  see also recipes
cookware, 149
coping techniques, 244-46
  see also relaxation
coronary artery disease, 7, 16
Coronary Drug Project, 23-24

D

depression, 60-63
diabetes, 53-57
diet, healthy, 89-91, 96, 109-11
  avocado, 123
  cilantro, 123
  eggs, 11, 53, 88
  fiber, 72-73
  fish, 80-81
  Mediterranean diet, 93-95
  pomegranate, 95-96

E

echium oil, 82-84
eggs, 11, 53, 88
emotional honesty, 241-44
endocarditis, 48
essential fatty acids (EFAs), 78-79
estrogen, 22-23
  and blood clotting, 29
  and brain function, 31-32
  and hormone replacement therapy
    (HRT), 23
  and magnesium, 30
exercise, 37-38
  overexercising, 206
  walking, 190, 191, 199
  weight training, 187-89, 190-94
  see also weight training program
exercises, 193-94, 217
  Bent One-leg Hip Lifts, 215
  Bridge with Leg Lifts, 200-201
  Cobras, 204-5
  Dips with Hip Lifts, 196-97
  Free Squat with Bicep Curl, 195-97
  Front Squat with 1/2 Shoulder
    Press, 208-9

  High Hip Lifts off Chair/Bench,
    207-8
  Knee to Opposite Elbow Bridge,
    211-12
  Lying Inner Thigh Leg Lifts, 204
  Moderate Range Windshield
    Wipers, 214
  Mountain Climbers, 209-10
  Push-ups, 198
  Side-to-Side Abdominal Twists, 216
  Side to Side Crunches with Legs Up,
    202-3
  Side-to-Side Stationary Lunges,
    206-7
  Skull Crushers in Hip Lift Position,
    210-11
  Squat "Ski Slope" Rows, 197-98
  Step Back Lunge with Bicep Curl,
    199-200
  Step-ups with Front Raises, 213
  Sumo Squats with Lateral Raises,
    201-2

F

family history, 32-33
fats, 73-74, 76, 85
  butter, 75
  coconut oil, 75-76
  echium oil, 82-84
  essential fatty acids (EFAs), 78-79
  flaxseed oil, 83-84
  omega-3 essential fats, 79-81
  saturated fats, 74-75
  trans fatty acids, 77
  unsaturated fats, 78
fiber, 72-73
fibrinogen, 45-46, 92, 184-85
fish, 80-81

fish oils see omega-3 essential fats

fitness see exercise

5-HTP (5-hydroxytryptophan), 66

flax meal, 114

flaxseed oil, 83-84

food see cooking; diet, healthy; recipes

Framingham Heart Study, 5, 6

free radicals, 12-13

   and pycnogenol, 172-73

fructose, 72

fruit, 72

G

gender, 20

ginger, 178

glucose see sugar (glucose)

glycation, 55-56

glycemic index, 70-71

H

Hay, Louise, 238

heart attack, 8, 13

   and anxiety attack, 65-66

   Monday factor, 16

   symptoms, 13-14, 15

heart disease, 5-7

   risk factors see risk factors for

      heart disease

heart failure, 16-17

   and Coenzyme Q10, 177

heart function, 7

heart health assessment, 105-8

HERS Trial, 24-25

high blood pressure (hypertension),

   50-51

   and Coenzyme Q10, 177

   and magnesium, 181

   and pycnogenol, 173-74

and sodium (salt), 99-100

high-density lipoprotein (HDL), 10, 41

homocysteine, 44

hormones, 21-22

   bioidentical progesterone, 27, 28

   and calcium and magnesium, 29-32

   hormone replacement therapy

      (HRT), 23

   synthetic hormones, 27, 28, 29

   see also estrogen

Hulley, Stephen B., 24

hypertension see high blood pressure

   (hypertension)

hypothyroidism see thyroid, low

I

imagery see visualization

inactivity, 37-38

inflammation, 47-48, 84

   and sytrinol, 169-70

insulin resistance, 54, 55, 74

iron (high levels), 45

ischemic heart disease, 7

K

Kuntz, Ted, 242-43

L

laughter, 239-41

lipoprotein(a) (Lp(a)), 43

low-density lipoprotein (LDL), 10, 11,

   41-42

M

magnesium, 99, 101-3, 179-81

   supplements, 180

   see also calcium and magnesium

meat, 90-91

meditation, 229-31
Mediterranean diet, 93-95
mercury contamination, 81-82
metabolic syndrome (syndrome X), 55
Miller, Dr. Michael, 240
myocardial infarction *see* heart attack

N
nattokinase, 92
negativity, 236-39
niacin, 183-85
Nurses Health Study, 80, 89-90
nutrients, 165, 185
    Coenzyme Q10, 175-79
    pycnogenol, 172-74
    sytrinol, 166-70, 172
    vitamins, 92-93, 181-85

O
obesity, 34-37
olive oil, 78
omega-3 essential fats, 79-81, 82-84
oral contraceptives, 30
    and smoking, 33
Ornish, Dr. Dean, 236
osteoporosis, 29, 31
Oz, Dr. Mehmet, 87

P
PEPI trial *see* Postmenopausal
    Estrogen/Progestin Interventions
    trial
pets, 63
PHASE Study, 25-26
plaque, 11, 13
pomegranate, 95-96
positive thinking, 237-39
Postmenopausal Estrogen/Progestin

Interventions trial, 27
potassium, 99-101
    and magnesium, 179
protein, 87-88, 89-91
    food sources, 89, 90
    meat, 90-91
    soy foods, 91-92
Provera, 28
pycnogenol, 172-74

R
recipes
    appetizers
        Black Bean Salsa, 123
        Breezy California Rolls, 124
        Eggplant Dip, 127
        Falafels in a Pita, 125
        Family Reunion Spinach Dip, 128
        Guacamole, 126
        Hummus, 127
        Seven-layer Mexican Party Dip,
            126
    breakfast
        Apple Oatmeal, 120
        Applesauce Surprise, 121
        Flax Pudding, 121
        Granola Crunch, 119
        Mom's Best Rice Pudding, 120
        Protein-packed Fruit Pudding, 119
        Rice Pancakes, 122
        Yogurt Shake, 122
    condiments
        Cheese-free Sauce with a Kick, 155
        Excellent Ginger Sauce, 155
        Quick and Easy Pesto, 157
        Tahini Sauce, 156
        Tzatziki (Cucumber Yogurt)
            Sauce, 156

desserts
    All-fruit Frozen Dessert (or
        Popsicles), 158
    Almond Butter Cookies, 162
    Apple Crisp, 159
    Blueberry Muffins, 160
    Herbed Biscuits, 158
    Snicker Snacker Instant Treats, 161
dressings
    Flax-vinegar Favorite, 129
    Lemon-garlic Dressing, 129
    Marvellously Easy Miso Dressing,
        130
    Multi-purpose Hearty Dressing,
        129
    Sweet Poppy Seed Salad Dressing,
        130
main dishes
    As Good As It Gets Pizza (Spelt
        Crust), 150
    Cauliflower Curry, 151
    Fassoulia (Beans), 152
    Fish with Zesty Orange Glaze, 154
    Herb-infused Halibut or
        Swordfish, 150
    Refried Beans (Frijoles Refritos), 152
    Southwest Chicken and Black
        Bean Pasta, 153
    Spicy Pepper Scallops, 154
salads
    Artichoke Greek Salad, 136
    Avocado and Sweet Nut Salad, 133
    "Catherine the Great" Salad, 133
    Marinated Broccoli and Cherry
        Tomato Salad, 132
    Mediterranean Tabouleh Salad, 135
    Mint-fresh Cucumber Salad, 135
    Shrimp and Sugar Snap Pea
        Salad, 134

    Spinach, Strawberry, and Feta
        Salad, 131
    Tofu Tempeh Salad with Curry, 131
soups
    Black Bean Soup, 138
    Classic Minestrone Soup, 141
    Dr. Ron's Vegetarian Chili, 144
    Lentil Carrot Soup, 139
    Ratatouille, 143
    Split Pea Sans Ham Soup, 142
    Traditional Japanese Miso Shi-ru
        with Vegetables, 137
    Traditional Tomato Soup, 140
spreads
    Better Butter, 163
    Coconut Butter-Flaxseed Spread,
        163
    Flax Egg Replacer, 163
    Mayonnaise, 164
vegetables
    Baked Spaghetti Squash, 146
    Fabulous Gingered Asparagus or
        Green Beans, 145
    Made-in-Minutes Sautéed
        Greens, 147
    Oil-less Vegetable Stir-Frizzle, 148
    Seasoned Broccoli Sauté, 146
    Thyme-to-Make Zucchini, 147
refined foods, 68, 69
relaxation, 223-24, 226
    deep breathing, 224-27
    laughter, 239-41
    meditation, 229-31
    visualization, 233-36
    yoga, 227-28
risk factors for heart disease, 19
    age, 19-20
    anger, 63-65
    apolipoprotein B (Apo B), 43

body shape, 38
C-reactive protein (CRP), 47-49
calcification, 92-93
depression, 60-63
estrogen levels, 22-27
and family history, 32-33
fibrinogen, 45-46
gender, 20
high blood pressure (hypertension),
   50-51
homocysteine, 44
hormone levels, 21-22
inactivity, 37-38
iron (high levels), 45
lipoprotein(a) (Lp(a)), 43
obesity, 34-37
smoking, 33
sugar (glucose), 53-56
thyroid, 20-21
triglycerides, 42-43
see also cholesterol

S

salt see sodium (salt)
Seelig, Dr. Mildred, 29, 30, 31, 180-81
selenium, 81-82
serotonin, 66, 69
Sircus, Dr. Marc, 81
smoking, 33-34
sodium (salt), 99-100
soy foods, 91-92
statins, 171, 175-77
stenosis see valve disorders
stress, 16, 219-23
   and the adrenal glands, 57-59
   and fibrinogen, 45-46
   and relaxation, 223-24, 226
stress test, 222-23

stroke, 179-80
sugar (glucose), 53-56, 68
   fructose, 72
   sugary beverages, 97
   sweeteners, artificial, 111-12
support networks, 62-63
surgery, preparing for, 228
sweeteners, artificial, 111-12
synthetic hormones, 27, 28, 29
sytrinol, 166-70, 172

T

tea, 98
thyroid, low, 20-21
trans fatty acids, 77
triglycerides, 42-43, 84
Type A personality, 64

U

unsaturated fats, 78

V

valve disorders, 15
VAP cholesterol test, 40, 43
very low-density lipoproteins (VLDL),
   39, 40, 42
visualization, 233-36
vitamins, 181-85
   vitamin K, 92-93

W

waist-to-hip ratio, 36-37
walking, 190, 191, 199
weight training, 187-89
   cardio options, 194
   core training, 191-93
   equipment, 190-91
   program outline, 193-94

warm-up, 194

see also exercises; weight training
   program
weight training program, 193-94, 217
   Day 1, 195-97
   Day 2, 197-99
   Day 3, 199-201
   Day 4, 201-3
   Day 5, 204-5
   Day 6, 206-8
   Day 7, 208-10
   Day 8, 210-12
   Day 9, 213-14
   Day 10, 215-16
Whitaker, Dr. Julian, 40
wine *see* alcohol consumption
Women's Health Initiative Study
   (WHI), 26-27, 28, 30
   and adverse cardiovascular effects,
      29
   and increase in mental decline, 31

Y

yoga, 227-28

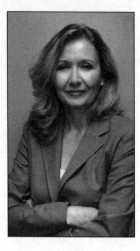

Lorna R. Vanderhaeghe, M.S., is Canada's leading women's natural health expert. Lorna has a Masters in Health Studies in nutrition and a degree in biochemistry. She is the author of thousands of articles and ten books, including *Sexy Hormones: Unlocking the Secrets to Vitality.* Lorna believes in empowering people with health knowledge so they may achieve optimal wellness. Lorna has an award-winning Web site, www.hormonehelp.com, and a free monthly health e-letter.

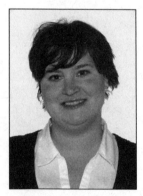

A graduate of the University of British Columbia School of Journalism with a specialization in alternative and complementary medicine, Michelle Hancock, M.J., has been writing about health and wellness for over ten years. To find out more about Michelle, visit www.michellehancock.ca

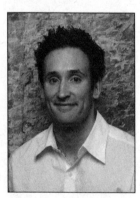

Byron Collyer, BSc., HKIN, is a certified personal trainer, high performance core specialist and internationally published health and fitness writer. He has written a women's weight loss manual tailored to the specific needs of women over 35. For more information on Byron, visit www.newedgehealth.com.